OCCASIONAL
P A P E R

Issues and Performance in the Pennsylvania Workers' Compensation System

Michael D. Greenberg, Amelia Haviland

 CENTER FOR HEALTH AND SAFETY IN THE WORKPLACE

A study by the RAND Institute for Civil Justice

The research described in this report was conducted within the RAND Center for Health and Safety in the Workplace (CHSW) with a grant from the Commonwealth of Pennsylvania.

Library of Congress Cataloging-in-Publication Data is available for this publication.

ISBN #978-0-8330-4408-2

The RAND Corporation is a nonprofit research organization providing objective analysis and effective solutions that address the challenges facing the public and private sectors around the world. RAND's publications do not necessarily reflect the opinions of its research clients and sponsors.

RAND® is a registered trademark.

Published 2008 by the RAND Corporation
1776 Main Street, P.O. Box 2138, Santa Monica, CA 90407-2138
1200 South Hayes Street, Arlington, VA 22202-5050
4570 Fifth Avenue, Suite 600, Pittsburgh, PA 15213-2665
RAND URL: http://www.rand.org/
To order RAND documents or to obtain additional information, contact
Distribution Services: Telephone: (310) 451-7002;
Fax: (310) 451-6915; Email: order@rand.org

Preface

Recent legislation in Pennsylvania, including a resolution in 2004 and a set of statutory reforms in 2006, suggest ongoing concerns about the performance and cost-competitiveness of the commonwealth's workers' compensation system. The purpose of this paper is to examine the performance of the system, identify some of the major policy issues that it faces, and describe potential options that the commonwealth might consider to address these issues. Focusing on benefits and compensation, safety, medical care, and dispute resolution, we draw on published data, where possible, to explore relevant performance benchmarks in these domains. Based on this analysis, we highlight several aspects of workers' compensation policy that will likely be prominent as targets for reform and more detailed empirical evaluation.

This study, which was sponsored by the Commonwealth of Pennsylvania, should be of interest to anyone who is concerned with workers' compensation policy in Pennsylvania, and particularly to policymakers interested in a broad perspective that spans several domains of performance within the system.

This research was conducted within the RAND Center for Health and Safety in the Workplace (CHSW) with a grant from the Commonwealth of Pennsylvania. CHSW is dedicated to reducing workplace injuries and illnesses. The Center provides objective, innovative, cross-cutting research to improve understanding of the complex network of issues that affect occupational safety, health, and workers' compensation. Its vision is to become the nation's leader in improving workers' health and safety policy.

The Center is housed at the RAND Corporation, an international nonprofit research organization with a reputation for rigorous and objective analysis on the leading policy issues of our time. It draws on the expertise within three RAND research units:

- RAND Institute for Civil Justice, a national leader in research on workers' compensation
- RAND Health, the most trusted source of objective health policy research in the world
- RAND Infrastructure, Safety, and Environment, a national leader in research on occupational safety.

The Center's work is supported by funds from federal, state, and private sources. For additional information about CHSW, please contact:

John Mendeloff, Director
Center for Health and Safety in the Workplace
RAND Corporation
4570 Fifth Avenue, Suite 600
Pittsburgh, PA 15213-2665
Email: John_Mendeloff@rand.org
Phone: (412) 683-2300, x4532; Fax: (412) 683-2800

Information about ICJ is available online (http://www.rand.org/icj/). Inquiries about research projects should be sent to the following address:

Robert T. Reville, Director
RAND Institute for Civil Justice
1776 Main Street, P.O. Box 2138
Santa Monica, CA 90407-2138
Email: Robert_Reville@rand.org
Phone: (310) 393–0411, x6786; Fax: (310) 451–6979

Contents

Figures

Tables

Summary

The workers' compensation system in Pennsylvania reflects a longstanding compromise between workers and employers, in which the former receive a guaranteed set of benefits in connection with workplace injuries and illnesses without regard to putative employer fault or negligence. In return, employers receive protection from tort liability regarding the same set of injuries. In principle, workers' compensation helps to provide certainty, both for workers and employers, in defining the parameters of liability for harms sustained in the workplace. Nearly 100 years after the adoption of the first workers' compensation laws by the states, however, modern workers' compensation systems involve complicated administrative mechanisms and standards for providing medical care to injured workers; for making difficult medical and legal determinations about the nature and treatment of occupational illnesses; for compensating workers' loss of income due to work-related disabilities; and for resolving disputes over claims through a channel removed from the ordinary judicial process. Notably, workers' compensation costs in many states have risen significantly over the last 30 years,[1] resulting in increasing financial pressure on employers and calls for systemic reforms. Consonant with the broader national pressures for reform, the workers' compensation system in Pennsylvania was the subject of major legislation in 1993 and 1996, and most recently again in 2006.

This paper was motivated by a legislative resolution in 2004 and the latest set of statutory reforms in 2006, which together suggest a continuing interest in costs and efficiency as drivers of workers' compensation policy in Pennsylvania. This paper examines some of the key policy issues that the Pennsylvania workers' compensation system faces and reviews available performance data from a number of sources. Our work focused particularly on surveying several aspects of the system: benefits and compensation, safety, medical care, and dispute resolution. In studying these aspects of workers' compensation policy, we undertook a broad review of available scholarly literature, performance data, and legal and regulatory materials concerning the Pennsylvania workers' compensation system (and to a much more limited extent, those of other states as well). To clarify and build on the results of our review, we also undertook a series of qualitative interviews with a range of stakeholder groups in the Pennsylvania system, including employers, officials, lawyers, physicians, and insurers. Based on the findings from our research, we identify a series of workers' compensation policies that may be prominent as targets for reform in the future, and we offer recommendations for addressing these issues through reform and additional performance assessment.

---

[1] Interestingly, costs to employers have declined on a national basis in the most recent available year of data, after several years of rising national costs during the early 2000s (Sengupta, Reno, and Burton, 2007, p. 84).

Overview of Performance and Policy in Pennsylvania

Several general observations emerge from a review of published data on benefits, cost, and compensation within the Pennsylvania workers' compensation system. First is simply the sense that Pennsylvania does not appear to be a system in crisis, or one in which employer costs are spiraling rapidly out of control. Although aggregate benefit payments in Pennsylvania are above the median when compared with those of other states, adjusted measures of total costs per claim (i.e., controlling for differences across states in injury and industry mix) suggest that the commonwealth is doing reasonably well compared with other states, and particularly so in regard to the rate of growth in costs over recent years. As mentioned above, Pennsylvania instituted a series of statutory changes to try to stem growth in workers' compensation costs during the 1990s. More recent data on benefits and costs (from 2000 to 2004) suggest that the earlier changes may have been successful in that aim. In contrast to the relatively abundant performance data that are available concerning payment levels, however, there are comparatively little data to address the questions of adequacy of indemnity benefits and how well the system actually does in replacing lost wages for workers who are seriously injured while on the job. Comparative interstate data for some other important measures of outcomes, notably speed of return-to-work, are also limited.

Promoting safety within the workers' compensation system has become a major priority for Pennsylvania policymakers, as reflected both by statutory reforms adopted in 1993 and by the more recent initiatives of the Bureau of Workers' Compensation and the WorkSAFE PA coalition. Occupational injury statistics published by the commonwealth suggest that rates of workplace injuries have fallen substantially during the last 15 years or so, from about 29 injuries per 1,000 workers in 1990 to between 15 and 18 injuries per 1,000 workers in 2005.[2] Data to support rigorous interstate comparisons of injury rates are limited, however, and several exploratory analyses undertaken by RAND on OSHA data suggest that Pennsylvania may not outperform several peer states on some measures of safety outcomes. Meanwhile, specific Pennsylvania policies intended to address workplace safety, particularly insurance incentives given to employers to adopt certified safety committees, have generated only limited performance data concerning their effectiveness. Consequently, the future prospects for improving workplace safety in the commonwealth may be tied less to specific policy reforms than to improved data collection and assessment of those reforms on a prospective, pilot basis.

Medical care is likely to be a crucial aspect of workers' compensation policy in the future, because related costs continue to climb both in Pennsylvania and across the nation. Notably, Pennsylvania's workers' compensation medical costs are relatively low, on a series of measures, compared with those of a number of other states. Comparative interstate data on access to care, health care quality, and worker outcomes are sparser, although the commonwealth has for many years conducted its own survey study looking at medical access and self-reported outcomes within the workers' compensation system. Prominent aspects of previous medical policy reforms already enacted in Pennsylvania include provider panel requirements, utilization review oversight, and a medical fee schedule based on Medicare circa 1994 (with subsequent annual adjustments based on state wage rates). Future reforms to further strengthen cost

---

[2] Although not directly comparable to Pennsylvania's numbers, national statistics from the Bureau of Labor Statistics Survey of Occupational Injuries and Illnesses suggest that the U.S. rate of nonfatal workplace injuries has also been on the decline since the early 1990s (Bureau of Labor Statistics, 2002, p. 16).

controls could build on any of these mechanisms, but, in any case, policymakers will need to balance considerations of cost containment against competing interests in maintaining access to care, quality of care, and good outcomes for injured workers. Given the skew in available performance data toward medical costs (and away from quality indicators), it would be easy for policymakers to focus inadvertently on the former set of concerns to the detriment of the latter.

Finally, dispute resolution within the workers' compensation system has also been the target of several major reforms in the last decade, including the institution of "compromise and release" (C&R) agreements in 1996 and the enactment of mandatory mediation requirements in 2006. Recent years of performance data suggest that the Pennsylvania Department of Labor and Industry's Office of Adjudication is now resolving workers' compensation cases more quickly and has reduced the backlog of cases within the system. On a complementary note, Pennsylvania does not appear to be an outlier when compared with a number of other states on several measures of litigation costs and litigiousness. This being said, the performance data that are currently available mostly focus on measures of litigation speed and cost, rather than on quality of outcomes or on the experience of litigants as participants in the justice system. As with workers' compensation medical care, future reforms on dispute resolution will need to balance considerations of cost against considerations of quality, both in outcomes and processes. Expanded efforts within the system to collect detailed outcome data on dispute resolution, particularly regarding initiatives such as mandatory mediation and compromise and release agreements, could provide new and useful insights to policymakers.

Key Observations and Recommendations

Based on the findings of our investigation into the workers' compensation system in Pennsylvania, we offer the following set of conclusions and recommendations for policymakers:

- Currently available data suggest that benefit payments in the Pennsylvania system, adjusted for payroll growth, have been relatively flat during 2000–2004, and that Pennsylvania compares favorably with a number of other states on several measures of average costs per workers' compensation claim. Far less clear is the adequacy of wage replacement associated with Pennsylvania's indemnity benefits and how well Pennsylvania compares to other states on this criterion. *Pennsylvania policymakers should consider the adequacy of wage replacement, as well as systemic payment levels, in assessing the overall performance of the system.* Either BWC or independent researchers should be encouraged to perform analyses on the adequacy of wage replacement in the commonwealth, so that policymakers can track and understand related trends over time.
- One of the most important reforms to the Pennsylvania system over the past 15 years was the institution of compromise and release agreements, which allow claimants and insurers to negotiate final, lump-sum settlements in discharge of workers' compensation liability. Nearly a third of the total benefits paid by the system in 2005 were disbursed through C&R agreements. Here again, though, the impact of C&R settlements on adequacy of wage-replacement benefits, long-term vocational outcomes, and medical care for injured workers is not well understood. *Ideally, the commonwealth should collect and aggregate more information about C&R agreements, who is entering into them, and what the major features*

of those agreements are. Future studies of wage-replacement adequacy in Pennsylvania should also look specifically at the impact of C&R, as compared with the traditional payment of claims. *Finally, any future proposals for additional C&R reforms, such as eliminating hearing requirements or mandating the existence of a genuine dispute between litigating parties, should be formally evaluated on a pilot or prospective basis.*

- New requirements for dispute mediation, instituted in 2006, are among the most recent reforms to the Pennsylvania system. Under the revised law, all workers' compensation claims that enter litigation must be mediated, except where a judge makes a finding on good cause that mediation would be futile. Given the newness of the requirements for mediation, however, there is currently no information on the effects of the mandate, on the nature and volume of cases resolved in the commonwealth through mediation, or on whether mediation produces materially different outcomes than adjudication across otherwise similar cases. *Pennsylvania stands in good position to track these kinds of measures going forward, and could thereby help policymakers in reviewing any future proposals to refine or expand on the current mediation requirements.*

- Rates of workplace injuries in Pennsylvania fell substantially between 1996 and 2005, according to aggregated workers' compensation data published by the commonwealth. Interstate comparisons of occupational injury rates are hampered, however, by differences in underlying definitions and methods for compiling data across the states. Notably, the Bureau of Labor Statistics (BLS) fields an annual Survey of Occupational Injuries and Illnesses, which estimates industry-specific injury rates both nationally and for 42 states, not including Pennsylvania. *The commonwealth should consider requesting that BLS increase its survey sample in Pennsylvania, so that comparable state-level injury rates will become available.*

- One of Pennsylvania's major initiatives to promote workplace safety involves encouraging employers to adopt certified safety committees, by providing a 5-percent discount on workers' compensation insurance premiums for participating employers. Uptake of certified safety committees within the employer community has been modest, however, and the limited safety performance data on the committees that are currently available through PCRB are only suggestive, but not conclusive, that the state certification program has had a beneficial effect. *Pennsylvania should seek better performance data to gauge the impact of certified safety committees on workplace injuries, as a precursor to any effort to expand the reach and influence of safety committees in the employer community.* More broadly, the commonwealth should consider new ways to make the financial benefits to employers of improved safety performance more transparent and more salient, throughout the employer community.

- Medical payments represent the part of aggregate workers' compensation payments that are growing most rapidly in Pennsylvania (and across the nation). And although Pennsylvania, when compared with a number of other states, has lower average medical costs on a per-claim basis, general trends toward growth in medical costs remain a subject of concern. Meanwhile, only limited performance data are currently being collected by the commonwealth describing quality of care and access within the Pennsylvania system, and interstate comparisons and benchmarking on those sorts of parameters are very limited. *Policymakers should continue to track measures of medical cost, and should improve the tracking of quality of care and access within the workers' compensation system, given that the pressures for medical cost containment are unlikely to diminish.*

- One aspect of the workers' compensation medical framework that has occasionally been criticized is the medical fee schedule, which in turn is based on the Medicare schedule from the early 1990s. Medicare fees have since been revised in ways not reflected by the Pennsylvania fee schedule, thereby giving rise to concerns about administrative burdens, as well as the potential for perverse incentives to providers that might undercut the aim of containing costs. We note that any proposed reform to the Pennsylvania fee schedule, particularly if intended to emulate current fee rates under Medicare, would likely involve highly technical details in the transition, as well as significant groups of winners and losers within the provider community. *As a precursor to any such proposal, we recommend that the commonwealth undertake a detailed study of the price implications of, and implementation options for, revising the medical fee schedule, along the lines of a similar assessment that was performed in California in 2003 (Wynn, 2003).*

- Pennsylvania has implemented several other important policies for containing workers' compensation medical costs since 1993, including provider panel requirements and utilization review oversight. Both of these mechanisms could be refined or expanded on in the future, and as of fall 2007, the commonwealth was reviewing a set of proposed regulations to update and clarify the current framework for utilization review. *We suggest that any future reforms to these policies incorporate a formal, prospective assessment of their ultimate effect on costs, as well as on health care quality and access.* This kind of performance information could help policymakers in evaluating the successfulness of the policies, as well as in refining them going forward.

Acknowledgments

The authors would like to thank the many stakeholder representatives in Pennsylvania who cooperated with the RAND research team to make their insights and perspectives available. We are also grateful to John Mendeloff and Robert Reville for their input and suggestions regarding our work. We would also like to acknowledge Asha Pathak, for her assistance in collecting and analyzing research materials, and Michelle Horner, for her patience and help in preparing this manuscript.

Abbreviations

BLS	Bureau of Labor Statistics
BWC	Pennsylvania Bureau of Workers' Compensation
C&R	compromise and release
CFOI	Census of Fatal Occupational Injuries
CPT	Current Procedural Terminology
DLI	Pennsylvania Department of Labor and Industry
LBFC	Pennsylvania General Assembly Legislative Budget and Finance Committee
NASI	National Academy of Social Insurance
ODI	OSHA Data Initiative
OSHA	Occupational Safety and Health Administration
PCRB	Pennsylvania Compensation Rating Board
PPD	permanent partial disability
SAWW	statewide average weekly wage
SIC	Standard Industry Classification code
SOII	Survey of Occupational Injuries and Illnesses
UR	utilization review
WCAB	Pennsylvania Workers' Compensation Appeals Board
WCRI	Workers Compensation Research Institute

CHAPTER ONE
Introduction

State workers' compensation systems involve a basic trade-off in risks affecting workers and employers, such that grievances over workplace injuries are removed from the civil justice system and dealt with through a no-fault administrative compensation scheme. The simple idea behind workers' compensation is to provide greater certainty and less risk, to both workers and employers, in redressing the consequences of workplace injury. Nearly a century following the adoption of the first workers' compensation laws by the states, however, the simplicity of the original premise has been overshadowed by complicated administrative mechanisms, pervasive adversarial interests, and fundamental tensions between competing policy goals.

Workers' compensation involves a number of major functions, each complex in itself, and each of which interacts with the others (see Figure 1.1). One of the major functions involves the delivery of health care services to workers. This function faces all the challenges involved in financing and utilization that plague the health care system more generally, as well as additional complications caused by the fact that medical providers in workers' compensation have relationships with employers as well as with workers.[1] Beyond medical benefits, workers' compensation also generates indemnity benefits for workers in order to redress the impact of temporary and permanent disability. In connection with claims for both medical and indemnity benefits, workers' compensation involves an administrative judicial framework for resolving disputes, in which litigation activity, costs, and speed of resolution play a major role in determining the effectiveness of the system for all parties. Finally, workers' compensation involves an elaborate set of standards and activities on the part of the states: promoting occupational safety, establishing fundamental rights for workers and requirements for employers, regulating the insurance and financial aspects of the systems, and in some instances placing the states directly into the market as insurers of workers' compensation risk. It should come as no surprise that several of these aspects of workers' compensation policy have been controversial over the years, as different states have adopted reforms to address rising costs and to modify the contours of no-fault compensation for workplace injuries.

The workers' compensation system in Pennsylvania has confronted many of the same challenges and historical issues that have arisen in other parts of the United States. In particular, concerns about rising workers' compensation costs in Pennsylvania led to a series of legislative reforms in the 1990s, a legislatively mandated study of the Pennsylvania system in 2004, and, most recently, an additional set of legislative reforms in 2006. The various reforms to the

---

[1] Medical care in workers' compensation involves some incremental functions for participating physicians, including the evaluation of permanent impairment and ability to return to work, as well as a corresponding set of administrative and paperwork burdens. Whether physicians are adequately compensated for these responsibilities under workers' compensation is a matter of open debate.

Figure 1.1
A Summary of the Major System Functions in Workers' Compensation

Safety and Injury Prevention

- Provide incentives and resources for promoting workplace safety
- Establish workplace safety standards and requirements
- Enforce safety requirements through inspections and penalties

Medical Care

- Provide post-injury treatment to workers
- Facilitate workers' recovery and return to work
- Evaluate worker injuries to determine eligibility for medical and indemnity benefits

Indemnity

- Evaluate worker injuries to determine eligibility for indemnity benefits
- Compensate lost income associated with temporary or permanent disabilities
- Assess any changes in disability status over time

Dispute Resolution

- Receive and hear petitions in disputed workers' compensation cases
- Resolve disputes over eligibility and benefit determinations
- Provide mediation and oversight for out-of-court settlements

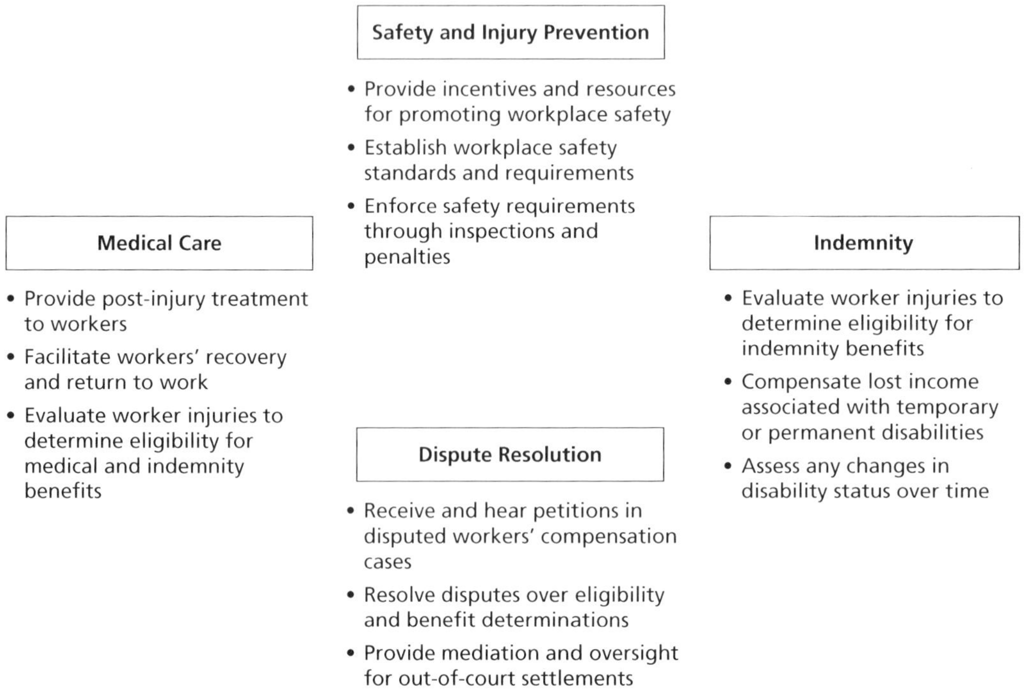

RAND *OP216-1.1*

Pennsylvania system have effected far-reaching changes to the medical, indemnity, and dispute resolution systems in the commonwealth. We briefly describe the history of these changes, and some of the major features of the Pennsylvania system, below. Note that the recent history of systemic reforms to the Pennsylvania workers' compensation system invites an evaluative question: How well is the system actually doing? One obvious criterion of performance is cost, including the extent to which the system appears to have stabilized following a period of growth in cost. Another criterion of performance is effectiveness: how well the various mechanisms and standards in workers' compensation continue to serve the purposes for which they were intended (e.g., in providing health care benefits, restoring lost income, making workplaces safer, etc.). One aim of this paper is to review available evidence on the performance of the workers' compensation system in Pennsylvania, addressing both of these criteria.

Workers' Compensation in Pennsylvania: Overview and Recent History

Participation in the workers' compensation system in Pennsylvania is compulsory for most private and public employers. Administrative responsibility for the system is divided between two agencies within the Pennsylvania Department of Labor and Industry (DLI): The Bureau of Workers' Compensation (BWC), which provides oversight for the safety, medical, claims management, and self-insurance functions of the system, and the Office of Adjudication, which carries out the judicial and dispute resolution functions. Under general guidelines established by the commonwealth, workers in Pennsylvania may be entitled to both medical and indemnity benefits in connection with their experience of workplace injuries and illnesses. Employers, meanwhile, are required to purchase insurance or to self-insure in order to pay for the benefits. In recent years, most workers' compensation benefits in Pennsylvania have been paid for through insurance contracts, although roughly 20 percent of benefits have been funded through employer self-insurance arrangements. Regulation of the financial aspects of workers' compensation is handled partly by Pennsylvania regulatory agencies (including BWC and the Department of Insurance) and partly by contract through the Pennsylvania Compensation Rating Bureau (PCRB). More detailed discussion of the structure of the Pennsylvania workers' compensation system, and of the processes by which claims actually pass through the system, are offered in the commonwealth's annual reports on workers' compensation (DLI, 2006b, 2007b). Additional characteristics of the system have also been described in several previous studies published by the Workers Compensation Research Institute (WCRI) (Telles, Wang, and Tanabe, 2006a, 2006d).

Prior to the 1990s, workers' compensation costs in Pennsylvania had undergone a period of substantial growth. Partly in response to concerns over the rising costs, the commonwealth passed a set of legislative reforms in 1993 entitled Act 44 (Commonwealth of Pennsylvania, 1993). Act 44 instituted a number of changes in the medical care aspects of the workers' compensation system, including (1) the establishment of a medical fee schedule based on then current Medicare reimbursement rates (with subsequent annual adjustment based on state wage rates); (2) formal mechanisms for utilization review (UR) in workers' compensation health care, with certification of corresponding UR organizations; and (3) the requirement that workers seek treatment through an employer-designated provider panel (if available) during the first 30 days following the occurrence of a workplace injury.[2] Act 44 also instituted a number of nonmedical reforms to the workers' compensation system, most notably by (1) allowing employers to pay benefits temporarily in the wake of an injury, without admitting any liability, and (2) enacting a series of new requirements regulating workers' compensation insurance arrangements and (separately) promoting health and safety in the workplace (Miller, 1994; Torrey and Greenberg, 2002).

A second set of reforms to the workers' compensation statute was enacted in 1996, pursuant to Act 57 (Commonwealth of Pennsylvania, 1996). The Act 57 reforms included additional modifications to medical care within the system, notably by extending the requirement for workers to seek treatment through their employers' provider panels (where available) during the first 90 days following the occurrence of an injury. Act 57 also included new provisions for administrative review of disputed medical fees, as well as some modifications in the rules concerning utilization review. More importantly, though, Act 57 also instituted major changes to the indemnity and dispute resolution aspects of the workers' compensation system. On the indemnity side, those changes included new requirements and standards concerning the assessment of permanent partial disability (PPD) status, establishment of a basic limit on the award of PPD benefits to no more than 500 weeks, and the imposition of new offset requirements for Social Security and pension benefits against workers' compensation disability benefits. On the dispute resolution side, Act 57 revised the standards for supersedeas proceedings (i.e., proceedings to modify or terminate benefits), in part by codifying a requirement for an administrative hearing prior to any modification in benefit payments, and in part by shifting the burden of proof in related hearings from employers to workers (DeBernardo, 1997). Perhaps most impor-

---

[2] Previously, the law had only required workers to seek treatment through provider panels during the first two weeks following injury.

tant, Act 57 established a "compromise and release" (C&R) procedure within the workers' compensation system, thereby allowing parties to negotiate final, lump-sum settlements in discharge of any obligations or benefits that would otherwise obtain. As one recent commentator pointed out, this single change in the law has had enormous impact on the workers' compensation system over the past ten years, with hundreds of millions of dollars in lump-sum payments now being issued pursuant to C&R agreements on an annual basis (Torrey, 2007).

Anecdotal accounts of costs in the Pennsylvania workers' compensation system suggest that those costs grew through the early 1990s, that the legislative reforms were intended to stem this growth, and that in fact the reforms may have been successful in doing so. Those anecdotes are borne out, at least in part, by published data. In a review of trends from 15 years of workers' compensation benefits data in Pennsylvania, the National Academy of Social Insurance (NASI) concluded that benefits paid (per $100 of covered payroll) grew by about 20 percent from 1989 to 1993. By contrast, between 1993 and 2001, the benefits paid (per $100 of covered payroll) fell by about 38 percent and then remained basically flat through 2004, the most recent year for which Pennsylvania data were available (Reno and Sengupta, 2006). Over the same 15-year period, the volume of workplace injuries in the commonwealth, and of workers' compensation indemnity claims, generally declined (Pennsylvania Compensation Rating Bureau, 2007). Detailed interpretation of these sorts of findings is complex, since the findings depend on underlying statistical methods, and were likely influenced by factors other than the Pennsylvania legislative reforms during the 1989–2004 time period. In particular, the NASI results are also noteworthy in showing that benefit payments *across the United States* followed a similar time trend as did those in Pennsylvania, with a pattern of rising payments through 1992 and then a long period of declining payments through 2000. Regardless, the published data are at least suggestive that patterns in workers' compensation benefit payments shifted in Pennsylvania after 1993, and that the shift occurred in close proximity to major legislative initiatives.

Notwithstanding these trends, the Pennsylvania General Assembly expressed continuing concern about the costs and efficiency of the Pennsylvania workers' compensation system in a legislative resolution in 2004 (Pennsylvania General Assembly, 2004). In that resolution, the assembly assigned its Legislative Budget and Finance Committee (LBFC) the task of conducting a comparative study of the Pennsylvania system and those of surrounding states. The LBFC study was published in 2005, and across a number of performance measures that were reviewed, suggested that the Pennsylvania system was not radically out of line with the performance of its peer states (LBFC, 2005). Where relevant in this paper, we touch on the earlier findings and recommendations of the LBFC study. For current purposes, though, it suffices to emphasize that the LBFC study reflected continuing legislative concerns about system performance and cost in Pennsylvania, even during a period of relative stability in aggregate levels of workers' compensation benefit payments and claims volume.

Most recently, the Pennsylvania legislature enacted still another set of workers' compensation changes through the passage of Act 147 in 2006 (Commonwealth of Pennsylvania, 2006b). Major reforms instituted under Act 147 included provisions for mandatory trial scheduling, resolution hearings, and mediation proceedings in workers' compensation litigation; the addition of a new set of rules governing the operation and membership of the Workers' Compensation Appeals Board (WCAB); and the establishment of an uninsured employers guaranty fund. Act 147 also included some additional provisions limiting attorney fees under compromise-and-release agreements; constraining assignment of cases to judges based on geography;

and raising the minimum compensation payment for injuries sustained prior to September 1993 to $100 per month. Of these various changes, the new requirements for trial scheduling, mediation proceedings, and expedited resolution hearings (to approve C&R agreements) are all aimed at improving the efficiency of workers' compensation adjudication mechanisms. Once again, these sorts of reforms highlight continuing interest in the speed with which the system resolves disputes over claims, and, by implication, in concerns about related costs. As of 2007, corresponding changes in the operation of the Office of Adjudication had been implemented only during the past year: It remains to be seen what the effects of the most recent round of legislative changes will actually be.

For current purposes, the recent history of the Pennsylvania workers' compensation system illustrates several things. First, the system is fundamentally dynamic and has continued to evolve over time. Second, concerns over costs remain a factor in the operation and evolution of the system. Third, many different aspects of workers' compensation policy have been the subject of change in the last 15 years, including dispute resolution and adjudication mechanisms, health care requirements and oversight, indemnity benefit structure, workplace safety initiatives, and insurance regulation and oversight. Taken together, these observations about the recent past suggest that the system will continue to change in the future. In particular, it seems likely that issues of cost within the system will continue to be a focus of interest and concern for at least some stakeholder groups; and likewise, that there are a number of aspects of workers' compensation policy that may invite further innovation or intervention in years to come.

Investigating Workers' Compensation Policy in Pennsylvania

The primary aim of this paper is to explore some of the major policy issues that the Pennsylvania workers' compensation system faces and to describe options that the commonwealth might consider in addressing these issues. As noted earlier, this paper also seeks to review available evidence on the performance of the system, based on published data. One of the basic attributes of the workers' compensation infrastructure is the extent to which data are available to assess the performance of the different functions of the system. Where we were unable to find or access relevant data in our research, we make note of that as well: One obvious target for future policy reform could be simply to upgrade data collection and processing efforts, so that policymakers in the future will have access to better and more complete information about how well the workers' compensation system is doing. Regardless, our main focus in this paper is on several specific aspects of the system, including benefits and employer costs, compensation and return to work, safety, medical care, and adjudication and dispute resolution. Although we do not address other elements of the system (particularly finance and insurance mechanisms) in detail here, we have nevertheless incorporated pertinent observations as these relate to our main topics of investigation.

The analysis in this paper is based on several different types of research activities. We started by conducting a background review of literature on the Pennsylvania workers' compensation system, drawing on historical, legal, and scholarly materials available through the Web and through topical databases including PubMed (medicine) and LexisNexis (law). We then focused on published data summaries and previous reports describing the performance of the system, from sources including the NASI, the WCRI, the PCRB, and the Pennsylvania

Department of Labor and Industry. Finally, we undertook a series of semi-structured interviews with a range of stakeholder experts to elicit feedback concerning policy issues related to the workers' compensation system, the performance of the system, and possible targets or options for future reform efforts. We endeavored to speak with representatives from a number of different stakeholder groups, including employers, insurers, workers' compensation physicians, lawyers (plaintiff- and defense-side), and government officials, in order obtain a broad set of perspectives on the system and the issues confronting it.[3] In all, we spoke with approximately 20 people, and with at least two or three persons from each group. Throughout this paper, we present relevant findings and insights from these interviews, without attribution of comments to specific persons.

In the remainder of this paper, we investigate and address a series of policy issues and options concerning the Pennsylvania workers' compensation system. Chapter Two provides an overview of trends in benefits paid, employer costs, and compensation and then examines the implications of those trends for policy. Chapter Three focuses on workplace safety programs and performance in connection with the mandates of the workers' compensation system. Chapter Four offers a review of the medical care aspects of the system, while Chapter Five undertakes a review of the dispute resolution mechanisms in the system. Finally, Chapter Six offers a discussion of some of the main implications gleaned from the analyses in preceding chapters and concludes with a list of key observations and recommendations for policymakers, across all of the areas of the Pennsylvania workers' compensation system that we studied.

---

[3]   We also endeavored to speak with representatives from several organized labor groups in connection with this study, but were ultimately unable to do so.

CHAPTER TWO

Benefits, Employer Costs, and Compensation

Any discussion of workers' compensation policy in Pennsylvania depends first on understanding some basic performance characteristics of the system as a context. What is the magnitude of benefits paid and costs associated with workers' compensation, how generously does the system compensate injuries, and how effective is it in returning injured claimants to work quickly? Measures of aggregate benefits paid and costs incurred offer a window into the size of the system, the magnitude of liabilities that it addresses, and how it has changed over time. System costs are particularly important to understand, in part because they reflect the underlying pressures for reform, as well as the effects of reforms already instituted. In this chapter, we draw on published data from several sources to describe Pennsylvania's performance on benefits paid, employer costs, and measures of compensation and return to work. Where possible, we examine trends in outcomes on these measures, as well as comparisons between Pennsylvania's experience and that of other states. In the final part of this chapter, we discuss some of the implications of findings on benefits, costs, and return to work, incorporating input that we received from our interviews with stakeholders about these topics.

Benefits and Employer Costs: Performance Data and Comparisons

There are a number of different methods and data sources for examining trends in workers' compensation costs in Pennsylvania. One of the simplest involves looking at aggregate annual benefits paid, which loosely reflects the most important element of costs to employers (setting aside other elements of cost, such as those uniquely attributable to insurance). The National Academy of Social Insurance has published extensive statistics describing total workers' compensation benefits paid per $100 of covered payroll, by state—a measure of aggregate benefits that facilitates interstate comparisons by adjusting for the effects of differences in population and wage levels across states.[1] According to NASI, Pennsylvania benefits paid per $100 of covered payroll were basically stable from 2000–2004 and averaged $1.28 per $100 of covered payroll per year, on an annual basis (see Figure 2.1). By comparison, over the same period, New York and the nation as a whole paid somewhat lower levels of benefits than did Pennsylvania, Ohio paid a similar level of benefits, and West Virginia paid a considerably greater level of benefits (which incidentally were the highest in the United States) (Sengupta, Reno, and Burton, 2006). In 2004, the most recent year for which NASI data are available, Pennsylvania ranked

---

[1] NASI combined information from several different sources in computing its state-by-state estimates of benefits paid, and employed different methods in calculating benefits for the insured and self-insured segments of the market. For discussion of methods details, see Sengupta, Reno, and Burton (2006, pp. 13, 75).

Figure 2.1
Workers' Compensation Benefits per $100 of Covered Wages

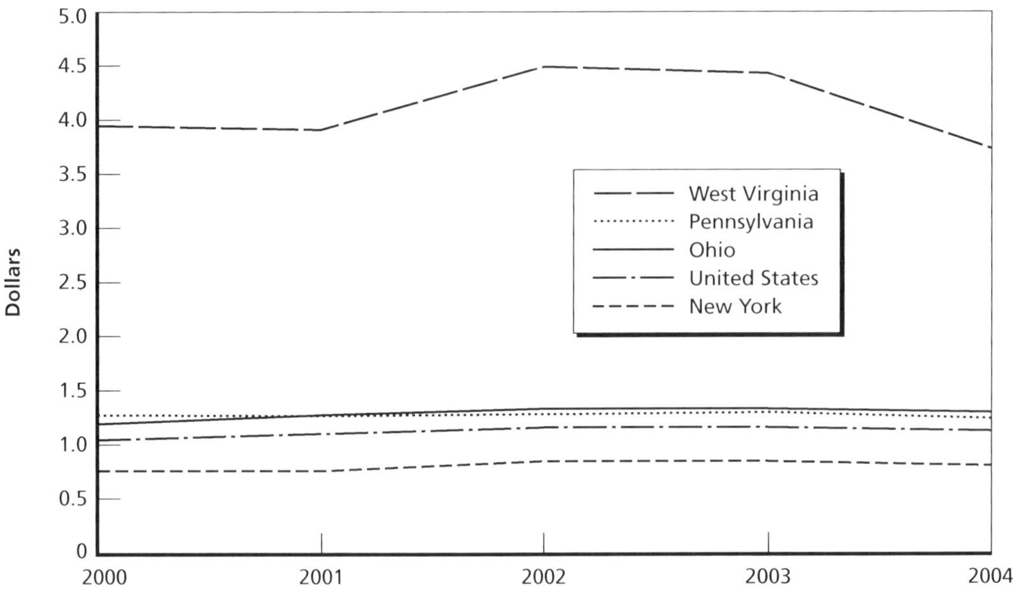

SOURCE: Abstracted from NASI statistics in Sengupta, Reno, and Burton, 2006.
RAND OP216-2.1

as the 13th-largest benefit payer among the 50 states and the District of Columbia, in terms of total annual benefits paid per $100 of covered payroll—a result that presumably reflects differences in the mix of industries and injuries, and in the generosity of benefit levels, across states. Note that we explore patterns in some of these explanatory variables in Chapter Three of this paper.

Another important set of measures on workers' compensation costs is available from statistics published by the Workers Compensation Research Institute (Telles, Wang, and Tanabe, 2006b, 2006d). In particular, WCRI studied workers' compensation in a group of 13 comparison states, including Pennsylvania, and computed a measure of average total cost per claim (for all paid claims), by state. Moreover, WCRI adjusted its measure of costs per claim to account for differences in injury mix, industry mix, and wage levels across states.[2] For claims that were incurred between October 2002 and September 2003 (and with costs evaluated as of early 2004), Pennsylvania had an average total cost per claim of $3,143, a result which was below the median for the 13 comparison group states ($3,450) and which ranked Pennsylvania as fourth-lowest in costs among them (Telles, Wang, and Tanabe, 2006a, 2006d). WCRI also tracked the time trend in growth of average total costs per claim[3] and found that Pennsylvania costs

---

[2]   The 13 WCRI comparison group states are Arizona, California, Florida, Illinois, Indiana, Louisiana, Massachusetts, Maryland, North Carolina, Pennsylvania, Tennessee, Texas, and Wisconsin. The WCRI measure of average total cost per claim includes both indemnity and medical benefit payments per claim, as well as benefit delivery expenses per claim. As with NASI's statistics, the WCRI statistics are compiled from a number of different data sources, and the technical methods by which the data were aggregated and adjusted are complex. For a detailed description of those methods, see Telles, Wang, and Tanabe (2006c, p. 68).

[3]   More precisely, WCRI analyzed the time trend in growth rates for average total cost per claim for all paid claims at 12 months' average maturity. See Telles, Wang, and Tanabe (2006d, p. 70).

grew by 7.4 percent annually, on average, between 1998 and 2004 (Telles, Wang, and Tanabe, 2006d). Interestingly, though, the growth in Pennsylvania's average total costs per claim consistently fell below the median value among the 13 comparison group states over the same time period. Taken together, these results suggest that employer costs per claim in Pennsylvania may compare favorably to those from a number of other states and that growth in those costs has been somewhat slower in Pennsylvania than elsewhere. WCRI has undertaken analyses on a series of additional measures of employer costs, focusing on different sets of claims (e.g., those involving more than seven days of lost work time) and on different components of cost. For the most recent available year of data, Pennsylvania appears to be at or below the median among the comparison group states on several different variations in these sorts of measures (Telles, Wang, and Tanabe, 2006d).

Beyond looking at simple measures of costs to employers, it can also be useful to track patterns in the major components of cost. For example, NASI has generated statistics on aggregate annual benefit payments by state, broken down by medical and indemnity benefits (Sengupta, Reno, and Burton, 2006). From 2000 to 2004, indemnity benefit payments in Pennsylvania grew by 3.6 percent (to approximately $1.53 billion), while medical benefit payments grew by 17.9 percent (to approximately $1.07 billion; see Figure 2.2). Remarkably, indemnity benefits across the entire United States grew by 11.6 percent, and medical benefits by 24.7 percent, during the same time period. These findings suggest that aggregate amounts of both medical and indemnity payments have grown more slowly in Pennsylvania than elsewhere in the country—importantly, this finding is not explained by differences in aggregate payroll growth, which rose by 12 percent in Pennsylvania and 10 percent across the United States over the same period of time (Sengupta, Reno, and Burton, 2006).

Figure 2.2
Aggregate Annual Workers' Compensation Benefits Paid in Pennsylvania, Medical Versus Indemnity

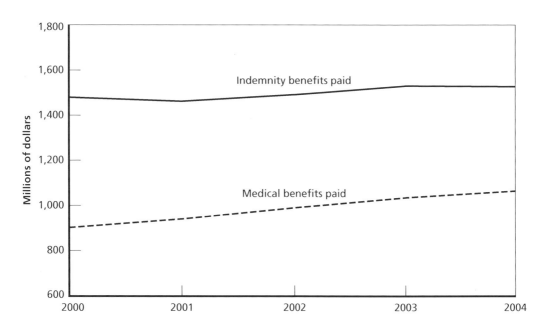

SOURCE: Abstracted from NASI statistics in Sengupta, Reno, and Burton, 2006.
RAND OP216-2.2

WCRI has also generated statistics breaking down the components of workers' compensation costs (indemnity benefit payments, medical benefit payments, and benefit delivery expenses) by state, on an average-cost-per-claim basis (for all paid claims).[4] As shown in Table 2.1, for the most recent available year of incurred claims (from October 2002 to September 2003), Pennsylvania's average cost per claim fell below the median values among the 13 comparison group states for indemnity payments, medical payments, and benefit delivery expenses (Telles, Wang, and Tanabe, 2006d).[5] A separate WCRI study looked at the comparative time trends in average medical payments per claim across states and found that Pennsylvania had the second-lowest rate of growth in medical costs among the comparison group states over the 1997–2002 period (Eccleston, Wang, and Zhao 2005b).

Finally, still another measure of workers' compensation costs to employers can be gleaned from insurance premium rates. Two separate studies of comparative insurance costs across the states were available from 2006. The Oregon Department of Consumer and Business Services published a premium rate–ranking study, based on data obtained from the National Council of Compensation Insurance (Reinke and Manley, 2006). That study created a composite manual rating of insurance premium costs for each state as of the end of 2005, based on the 50 most important industrial classifications in Oregon and then weighted by the industry mix in Oregon (to standardize for differences in industry mix across states). According to results from that study, the premium rate index for Pennsylvania was calculated at $2.80 per $100 in covered payroll, thereby placing the commonwealth at 113 percent of the median level of state premium-rate indices across all U.S. states. Based on this work, Pennsylvania was ranked as the 18th most expensive state in the nation, moving upward from 20th place in an earlier 2004 ranking (Oregon Department of Consumer and Business Services, 2005; Reinke and Manley, 2006). In a separate study that used a somewhat different set of methods and assumptions for computing state insurance premium rates (again as of the end of 2005), the average manual insurance rate for Pennsylvania was calculated at $4.53, which was reportedly 8 percent greater than the countrywide average manual rate and ranked the commonwealth as the 20th most expensive state (from among 45 states that were studied) (Actuarial and Technical Solutions,

Table 2.1
WCRI Average Total Costs per Claim, 2003–2004

Type of Claim	Pennsylvania's Average Cost per Claim	13-State Median, Average Cost per Claim	Pennsylvania Rank
Indemnity	$1,037	$1,295	4th
Medical	$1,725	$2,111	3rd
Benefit Delivery Expenses	$377	$410	6th

SOURCE: Abstracted from Telles, Wang, and Tanabe, *CompScope Benchmarks for Pennsylvania, 6th Edition*, Cambridge, Mass.: Workers' Compensation Research Institute, 2006.

---

[4] "Indemnity benefit payments," "medical benefit payments," and "benefit delivery expenses" are each specifically and formally defined by WCRI, in a way that corresponds with the underlying data that they collected for each measure. Detailed definitions and discussion of data and statistical methods are provided in Telles, Wang, and Tanabe (2006c, p. 68).

[5] WCRI data on workers' compensation payments are limited only to claims that were incurred during 2002–2003. By contrast, the NASI statistics on workers' compensation payments are not similarly limited to a narrow window of incurred claims. One practical implication of the difference is that the WCRI statistics omit long-term indemnity payments for injuries that occurred prior to 2002, whereas the NASI statistics include such payments. Consequently, it makes sense that NASI statistics suggest that aggregate indemnity payments exceed aggregate medical payments in Pennsylvania (Figure 2.2), even though WCRI statistics on average costs per claim superficially suggest the opposite (Table 2.1).

Inc., 2006). Note that interpretation of these sorts of insurance premium findings is difficult and requires caution, because both studies involved elaborate statistical methods and calculations not fully explained in the source reports.

In sum, what kind of composite picture of workers' compensation benefits and employer costs do we put together from these various sources? Clearly, aggregate levels of benefits paid (both medical and indemnity) have been climbing in Pennsylvania over the 2000–2004 time period and, in the most recent available year, were somewhat above the median value for other states.[6] Nevertheless, aggregate benefits paid appeared to be growing more slowly in Pennsylvania than in the nation as a whole: In other words, other parts of the country may be getting closer to Pennsylvania on this criterion. Per NASI statistics for 2004, Pennsylvania is striking both for paying an above-average level of benefits per $100 in covered payroll and for devoting a lower fraction of its workers' compensation benefits to medical care, as compared with most other states (Sengupta, Reno, and Burton, 2006). Taken together, these NASI results suggest that total indemnity benefits paid in Pennsylvania may be above average relative to other states. Findings from an independent study on workers' compensation benefits in 2002 are consistent with this proposition, showing that average temporary and permanent disability payment levels in Pennsylvania rank the commonwealth as one of the highest-paying states in the nation (Blum and Burton, 2006). Nevertheless, Pennsylvania ranked low in the frequency of claims that actually received permanent partial disability benefits, with relatively few injured workers obtaining such benefits. These results suggest that it may be comparatively difficult for workers to qualify for PPD in Pennsylvania, but that the benefit levels for those who do qualify may be relatively generous.

Looking at employer costs on an average per-claim basis, as in the WCRI findings, offers a more sophisticated and comprehensive way for making direct comparisons of workers' compensation costs across states (and adjusting for differences in industry mix, injury mix, and state payrolls). Notably, Pennsylvania showed relatively low costs on several of these measures and, in the most recent year, was below the median value for comparison group states on all components of cost. Although the time trends on the WCRI measures show that average total costs per claim in Pennsylvania have grown each year over the last five years, the rate of growth has nevertheless fallen below the median value for comparison group states throughout the time period—a finding that seems consistent with the pattern in growth of aggregate benefits paid described by NASI. Lastly, results from studies of insurance rate premiums are more difficult to interpret (because of underlying questions about methods and technical details) but superficially suggest that measures of aggregate insurance premium rates in Pennsylvania may be a bit higher than the median values across all other states.

Compensation and Return to Work: Performance Data and Comparisons

Beyond examining benefit payments and costs associated with the Pennsylvania workers' compensation system, it is also instructive to understand some basic parameters regarding indemnity payments within the system, including the typical length of time that disabled workers receive indemnity benefits (which can also be understood as a measure of return to work), the

---

[6]   Incidentally, the volume of claims and the size of the state's aggregate payroll during the same period were also above the median for other states.

maximum benefits available under the system, and the frequency with which workers receive permanent partial disability payments. In part, these sorts of parameters describe the basic generosity of indemnity benefits available through the system, as well as its effectiveness in getting injured claimants back to work quickly. They also offer a basis for comparing performance across states, not on cost, but rather on the nature of compensation benefits and (to some degree) the successfulness of the different systems in preventing or mitigating longer-term partial disabilities. The basic legal contours for compensation in the Pennsylvania system allow for an initial period of up to two years from the date of workplace injury, during which a claimant may be entitled to temporary total disability benefits at two-thirds of the claimant's pre-injury wage rate (subject to a statewide "maximum wage"). After two years of such temporary payments, a claimant then becomes obligated to undergo medical evaluation in order to receive continuing benefits. A finding of total permanent disability (based on a rating of greater than 50 percent impairment, per the American Medical Association's (AMA's) *Guides to the Evaluation of Impairment* [Cocchiarella and Anderson, 2001]) can lead to continuing payments on an indefinite basis, while a finding of partial permanent disability leads to payments for up to an additional 500 weeks, at a rate that is based either on a schedule for specific types of injuries (e.g., amputations) or else at two-thirds of the difference between the claimant's pre-injury wage rate and post-injury earning power.[7] Even after a claimant has been judged eligible for PPD benefits, changes in his or her employment or medical status can give rise to renewed evaluation of eligibility and level of continuing benefits.

WCRI has analyzed and published data concerning the duration of indemnity benefits among three "wage-loss" states—Pennsylvania, Louisiana, and Massachusetts—within its comparison group of states (Telles, Wang, and Tanabe, 2006b).[8] For claims arising between October 2002 and September 2003 (and evaluated as of early 2004), the average duration of temporary disability claims in Pennsylvania was 14 weeks, compared with 13 weeks in Massachusetts and 17 weeks in Louisiana (Telles, Wang, and Tanabe, 2006b).[9] Drawing on the same set of claims data, the fraction of claims (involving at least seven days of lost work time) that ultimately gave rise to PPD or lump-sum payments was 9 percent in Pennsylvania, 10 percent in Massachusetts, and 12 percent in Louisiana. These findings were broadly explained in terms of the structural difference between a "wage-loss" framework for PPD benefits (which compensates unscheduled injuries based solely on loss of earnings capacity) versus a "non-wage-loss" framework for PPD benefits (which compensates unscheduled injuries based on ratings of functional impairment).[10] WCRI advances the hypothesis that a wage-loss framework may create incentives for longer periods of temporary disability, because qualification for PPD benefits will tend to be more difficult than it would be in a non-wage-loss framework (Telles, Wang,

[7] See 77 Pa. Cons. Stat. Ann. § 511 et seq. (Commonwealth of Pennsylvania, 2007b).

[8] A "wage-loss" state is one in which indemnity benefits for permanent impairments that are not specifically included on a defined schedule are contingent on an actual loss of wages or earning capacity.

[9] As with other WCRI analyses described earlier in this chapter, results were adjusted to compensate for differences in industry mix, injury mix, and wage levels across states.

[10] Most (if not all) states have a workers' compensation "schedule" that determines indemnity benefits for a list of defined permanent disabilities—e.g., loss of an arm, loss of an eye, etc. For other forms of disability not specifically included on such a schedule, a small number of "wage-loss" states (including Pennsylvania) determine compensation based on continuing demonstrated loss of earnings capacity. By contrast, many other states determine compensation for unscheduled injuries based on a medical assessment of functional impairment, per standards established by the AMA's *Guides to the Evaluation of Permanent Impairment* (Cocchiarella and Anderson, 2001).

and Tanabe, 2006d)—a hypothesis that is at least not inconsistent with other published data showing that Pennsylvania has a relatively low frequency of PPD awards compared with other states, but comparatively high frequency and benefit levels with regard to temporary disability awards (Blum and Burton, 2006). Unfortunately, statistics comparing the duration of temporary benefits across wage-loss versus non-wage-loss states are not available through WCRI. Interestingly, though, we did find that Oregon independently reports on the average number of temporary disability days that were paid within that state per disabling claim, on an annual basis. Although not directly comparable to the WCRI statistics on Pennsylvania, the Oregon measure for duration of wage-loss benefits was 60 days (or 8.6 weeks) in 2003 (Oregon Department of Consumer and Business Services, 2006)—a result that is at least not contradictory to the idea that non-wage-loss states may tend toward shorter duration in temporary indemnity benefits (and by implication, in time away from work).[11]

With regard to legal standards for defining maximum indemnity benefits payable, Pennsylvania again permits compensation of up to 66.7 percent of an injured worker's wages in total disability benefits, provided that this amount does not exceed the statutory maximum compensation payable (which is set at 66.7 percent of the statewide average weekly wage [SAWW]).[12] Death benefits in Pennsylvania depend on the wages of the decedent and the nature and number of survivors: For example, benefits are set at 51 percent of the decedent's wages, capped at the SAWW, for a childless widow; 32 percent of wages, capped at the SAWW, for an orphaned single child; and 60 percent of wages, capped at the SAWW, for a widow with a single child.[13] For purposes of comparison, Table 2.2 shows the statutory limits on maximum indemnity compensation across several additional states, including New York, Ohio, and West Virginia. The results generally suggest that there is a lot of similarity across these states in the

Table 2.2
Maximum Indemnity Benefits by State, Selected State Comparisons

State	Maximum Indemnity Benefit	Maximum Death Benefit
Pennsylvania	66.7% SAWW	51% of decedent's wages for childless widow
		60% of decedent's wages for widow with single child
		32% of decedent's wages for an orphaned single child[a]
New York	66.7% SAWW	66.7% of decedent's wages allocated among widow and children (post-1978), subject to offsets for Social Security[b]
Ohio	66.7% SAWW	66.7% of decedent's wages apportioned among survivors[a]
West Virginia	100% SAWW	66.7% of decedent's wages apportioned among survivors, up to statutory cap of 100% SAWW

SOURCE: Compiled from relevant statutory provisions in Pennsylvania, New York, Ohio, and West Virginia.
[a] In all cases, wage levels are capped at SAWW.
[b] Specific caps on wage levels set by statute based on year of death.

---

[11] However, Oregon imposes only a three-day waiting period to qualify for temporary disability benefits, in contrast to the seven-day waiting period that applies in Pennsylvania—another reason why we might expect to see a shorter average duration of temporary disability benefits in Oregon as compared with Pennsylvania.

[12] See 77 Pa. Cons. Stat. Ann. § 25.1, 511 (2007).

[13] See 77 Pa. Cons. Stat. Ann. § 561, 562, 581 (2007).

formulas by which maximum indemnity benefits are capped, although West Virginia demonstrates that at least some states have chosen to institute their caps at a level higher than 66.7 percent of SAWW. The results also show that caps on benefits are basically tied to state average wage rates and therefore will be higher in states with higher wages. Finally, with regard to death benefits, the results suggest that the details of apportionment vary by state and are complex but that Pennsylvania's benefits may be set somewhat more restrictively than those in a number of other states. WCRI has also published a more detailed summary of PPD benefit formulas and statutory caps for its 13 comparison group states (Telles, Wang, and Tanabe, 2006a).

These kinds of characteristics and results with regard to indemnity benefits and compensation give some flavor for the Pennsylvania system. Although it pays out relatively high levels of aggregate benefits compared with other states, the indemnity benefit in Pennsylvania is nevertheless capped at two-thirds of the statewide average wage rate: Like many other states, Pennsylvania has made a basic policy decision not to fully compensate lost income associated with total disability for high-wage workers. Unfortunately, our discussion of compensation levels here provides only a very limited basis for comparing Pennsylvania to other states on speed of return-to-work following injury, a measure that is associated with the effectiveness of the system in helping injured workers to get back on the job quickly.[14] Perhaps more important, available statistics on indemnity benefits and temporary disability touch only indirectly, if at all, on the question of adequacy of benefits: Namely, how well do indemnity benefits within the state do in actually replacing lost income among injured workers with partial disabilities? A recent literature review on this point described results from a NASI analysis that found that Pennsylvania benefits for temporary total disability in 1998 were the most generous of any U.S. state (Hunt, 2003/2004). With regard to PPD benefits, several studies have looked at the issue of adequacy of benefits by estimating actual losses of income to injured workers. These studies examined adequacy of wage replacement across a small group of states, not including Pennsylvania (Reville et al., 2001, 2005). A similar investigation assessing the adequacy of benefits in the commonwealth could provide useful information to policymakers, by complementing the (relatively abundant) information that is already available about system costs.

Discussion and Policy Implications

Several general observations emerge from a review of published data on benefits, cost, and compensation within the Pennsylvania workers' compensation system. First is simply the sense that Pennsylvania does not appear to be a system in crisis, or one in which benefit payments and employer costs are spiraling out of control. Although aggregate benefit levels are fairly high relative to those of other states, adjusted measures of costs per claim suggest that Pennsylvania is doing reasonably well, and particularly so in regard to the growth in costs over recent years. As discussed earlier, Pennsylvania instituted a number of statutory reforms to try to stem growth in costs during the 1990s; the more recent data on benefits and costs (from 2000 to 2004) suggest that the earlier reforms may have been successful in their aim. Second, Pennsylvania's system reflects some fundamental policy choices about the nature and basis of

[14] Note, however, that WCRI performed a survey study in 2003 that addressed the question of speed of return-to-work in Pennsylvania relative to several other states. See Victor, Barth, and Liu (2003). We revisit the issue of return-to-work and discuss relevant survey results in Chapter Four, which discusses medical care in the Pennsylvania system.

compensable injuries. For example, the fact that Pennsylvania is a "wage-loss" state means that determinations of PPD status will often turn on demonstrated loss of earnings capacity rather than on ratings of functional impairment. Without commenting on the advantages and drawbacks of this kind of policy, it clearly has implications both for compensation within the system and for the kinds of evaluation and review tasks that the system will typically be called on to perform. Third, the types of performance data that are currently being collected and published by WCRI, NASI, and others provide a fairly detailed picture of benefits paid and costs accrued by the system. In contrast, there is comparatively little information available on adequacy of indemnity benefits and how well the system actually does in replacing lost wages and earnings capacity for workers who are seriously injured while on the job.

These observations are generally consistent with the comments we received during our interviews with stakeholders (particularly employers, insurers, and lawyers from both sides of the workers' compensation bar) in response to open-ended questions about benefit levels, costs, and compensation in Pennsylvania. Several people told us that the statutory reforms of the 1990s had basically been successful in stemming the growth of workers' compensation costs, but that costs nevertheless continue to rise, and that employers continue to be legitimately concerned about managing those costs effectively. Some interviewees also expressed uncertainty about the adequacy of indemnity benefits in replacing lost wages, particularly for workers who suffer long-term disabilities. Interestingly, we heard several comments about more specific concerns about cost drivers within the system. Regarding fraud (i.e., the filing of bogus or exaggerated claims for workers' compensation benefits), for example, several people suggested to us either that fraudulent claims within the system are not a major problem or that the incidence of fraud within the system had dropped in recent years, particularly in the wake of anti-fraud reforms that were enacted as a part of Act 44 in 1993. On the other hand, we also heard the view that there are always a handful of claimants who are looking to take advantage of the system in obtaining indemnity benefits, and that from an employer perspective, problems particularly arise in connection with claims based substantially on psychiatric injuries and traumatic stress. On a different issue, stakeholders expressed concerns about the 2006 reform (part of Act 147) that raised minimum indemnity benefit payments to $100 per week in cases of total disability based on pre-1994 injuries. Although the size of this increase in benefits is modest and is reimbursed by the state, it nevertheless raises the possibility of additional increases in indemnity benefits in the future, a prospect that elicited apprehension for one of the employers with whom we spoke.

In the remaining chapters of this paper, we focus in more depth on several aspects of workers' compensation policy and cost drivers, including safety, medical care, and dispute resolution within the system. For current purposes, it may suffice to note that benefit levels and employer costs are likely to continue to be a focus of attention and concern. And, as reflected in the comments from the stakeholders we interviewed, there is clearly a fundamental conflict between employers and workers over benefit levels and corresponding costs. At the same time, though, that conflict might also serve as a lever in further efforts to improve the system: namely, by focusing on those aspects of workers' compensation policy where the interests of employers and workers are well aligned, rather than in tension with each other.

CHAPTER THREE

Safety

Workers' compensation is a no-fault system for addressing the sequelae of workplace injuries by providing claimants with medical care and compensatory payments for their lost wages. Because employers are compelled to pay for the benefits to workers that are thus provided, there is a basic conflict of interest between employers and workers over the extent and applicability of those benefits. Employers and workers tend to have legitimate disagreements over a number of aspects of workers' compensation policy, including some of the primary contours that define indemnity and medical payments under the system. Presumably, though, all parties would agree that workplace injuries are a bad thing and that, in the abstract, preventing such injuries is desirable. For workers, the advantages to preventing injuries through improved workplace safety are clear. At best, workers' compensation is unlikely to compensate fully all of the harms associated with serious injury and lasting disability, so workers will always be better off by avoiding such injuries than by being compensated for them after the fact. Employers also stand to gain. Reductions in injuries have the potential to reduce compensation costs and, ultimately, insurance rates—an end that could be particularly attractive to employers, to the extent that the savings outweigh marginal investments in safety programs. Prevention of workplace injuries could also help employers avoid an additional set of costs unrelated to workers' compensation, including potential losses in labor and productivity, regulatory and compliance burdens, and reputational effects (both inside and outside the workplace). In essence, then, workplace safety is theoretically very attractive as a lever in workers' compensation policy because, other factors held equal, all parties would agree that the best system is one in which no worker ever gets hurt on the job.

This chapter provides a summary review of safety policies, and of evidence of performance concerning safety outcomes pertaining to the Pennsylvania system. Whereas in Chapter Two we discussed how workers' compensation costs in Pennsylvania have changed over time and how they compare to those of other states, here we shift focus to concentrate on the events and environments that give rise to those costs. In the remainder of this chapter we briefly describe the landscape of safety regulations and policies that apply in Pennsylvania. We then review some major findings from published studies and data on injury/illness rates in the commonwealth, and we also provide some new analyses, drawing on available injury data. We conclude with a discussion of some of the recent safety policy initiatives that have been implemented in Pennsylvania, what is currently known about the their effectiveness, and what insights can be gleaned about possibilities for future policy changes on workplace safety.

Summary of Workplace Safety Regulation and Policies in Pennsylvania

Decisions made by employers about workplace safety practices do not occur in a vacuum, but rather in the context of several existing sources of legal safety rules and mandates, some of them entirely outside the scope of the Pennsylvania workers' compensation system. Most broadly, pursuant to the federal Occupational Safety and Health Act of 1970 (P.L. 91-596), virtually all employers in the commonwealth have long operated under the mandate of an extensive set of health and safety regulations. These federal rules are enforced by the U.S. Occupational Safety and Health Administration (OSHA), which administers an inspection program to ensure compliance with federal standards. OSHA enforcement includes programmed (random) inspections, as well as targeted inspections to investigate complaints received against specific employers. OSHA inspections can focus on safety hazards, health hazards, or on both sets of concerns. These inspections can result in employers being cited for violations, which in turn can trigger a range of possible consequences, including federal fines and penalties. Consequently, OSHA regulations represent a serious set of workplace safety obligations for firms, despite the fact that the regulations are frequently complex and often burdensome to comply with. Although the commonwealth has no direct role in OSHA regulation or enforcement, it does join OSHA in providing financial support to an independent consultation program for employers: one that offers advice on OSHA compliance to small firms free of charge.[1]

Independent of federal workplace safety guidelines under OSHA, the Pennsylvania workers' compensation system also includes provisions specifically dedicated to promoting safety in the workplace. In connection with Act 44, in 1993 the legislature enacted a series of mandates for workers' compensation insurers and self-insured employers to provide accident- and illness-prevention services, as a prerequisite for their own state certifications. Details regarding the specific nature of accident-prevention services that are required in any particular business context are not defined by the statute, but in general the mandated services include "surveys, recommendations, training programs, consultations, analyses of accident causes, industrial hygiene and industrial health services."[2] In connection with providing these services, both insurers and self-insured employers are required to make available "qualified accident and illness-prevention personnel," in accordance with regulations promulgated by the Pennsylvania Department of Labor and Industry. The statute also authorizes DLI to conduct periodic enforcement inspections to ensure the adequacy of accident-prevention services under the workers' compensation system, and insurers and self-insured employers in the commonwealth are further required to submit detailed information about these services to DLI on an annual basis. Failure to comply with the accident-prevention requirements of the workers' compensation laws constitutes a civil violation and is punishable by fines of up to $2,000 per day.

In addition to the legal requirements for accident-prevention services, Act 44 also instituted a new incentive for employers to form voluntary safety committees and to seek formal certification of those committees from DLI: In return for doing so, employers are entitled to receive a statutory 5-percent discount in the premium rates for their workers' compensation insurance policies.[3] In connection with the statute, the state subsequently promulgated regula-

---

[1]   See Indiana University of Pennsylvania (undated) for a description of this program.

[2]   See 77 Pa. Cons. Stat. Ann. § 1038.1 (Commonwealth of Pennsylvania, 2007c).

[3]   See 77 Pa. Cons. Stat. Ann. § 1038.2 (Commonwealth of Pennsylvania, 2007d). Employers who self-insure are required to establish and maintain a safety committee as a condition of self-insurance, and they do not receive the 5-percent credit

tions describing in detail the membership, training, and operating requirements for certification of safety committees in Pennsylvania. In general, these committees need to include both worker and employer representatives; to meet at least on a monthly basis; to conduct workplace inspections designed to locate and detect health and safety hazards; and to review safety complaints and incidents involving work-related deaths, injuries, and illnesses.[4] Since 1993, the length of time over which employers are entitled to receive an insurance discount in return for maintaining their certified safety committees has been modified more than once, but at present the insurance discount is open-ended, subject to annual re-verification by employers that their safety committees remain active and fully compliant with the commonwealth's regulatory requirements.

Beyond these sorts of safety mandates and incentives as established by federal and Pennsylvania laws, there are also several other workplace safety activities and programs that are being orchestrated by the commonwealth. The Pennsylvania Bureau of Workers' Compensation, in particular, offers a number of safety-related services and resources to the employment community, in an effort to promote and improve local workplace safety efforts undertaken by employers and their workers. Perhaps most important, BWC activities include offering an extensive set of workplace safety training seminars in various parts of the commonwealth, on topics that are relevant for many different types of employers. BWC also offers support to employers through access to written materials on workplace safety, technical guidance, and standardized forms, as well as by providing information to employers about safety professionals resident within the state. BWC has recently been involved in an initiative to upgrade its connection to the employment community via a new Web-based portal called "HandS," which is designed to support electronic filings and data interchange and may facilitate both improved data collection by the bureau and improved dissemination of safety information and training opportunities to employers (DLI, 2007a).

Outside the formal regulatory aegis of BWC, another important public-private partnership is also seeking to promote workplace safety in the commonwealth. In recent years, the governor's administration, in conjunction with the Department of Labor and Industry, created an umbrella workplace safety initiative called "WorkSAFE PA" (DLI, 2007d). This initiative includes an advisory board with stakeholder representatives from labor, industry, and government; an annual conference for the employment community on workplace safety; and the creation of a "Governor's Award for Safety Excellence," a competitive honor that is designed to provide information about best practices in workplace safety, in addition to recognizing employers and their employees who demonstrate safety excellence. WorkSAFE PA serves as a community platform for exchanging information on workplace safety and for providing technical assistance to employers. One prominent example of WorkSAFE PA's technical support involves a set of online resources that were developed to assist employers in establishing internal "Return-to-Work" programs (DLI, 2007c), with the purpose of facilitating the safe return of injured workers to modified employment. Related resources walk an employer through all the steps needed to create and operate such a program, complete with numerous sample forms, documents, and presentations appropriate for all relevant stakeholder groups.

---

for having done so.

[4] See 34 Pa. Code § 129.1005 (Commonwealth of Pennsylvania, 2007a). Certified safety committees are subject to a number of additional requirements and operating responsibilities, beyond those listed above.

The foregoing summary illustrates that there are many applicable legal rules, standards, and activities pertaining to workplace safety currently in effect in Pennsylvania. Some of the relevant laws and programs are expressly based in the commonwealth and closely tied to the operation of the workers' compensation system; others involve broader state or federal authority and affect the workers' compensation system only incidentally. In the next section of this chapter, we describe general results concerning workplace safety performance in Pennsylvania. The most important question to address, though, is how effective any of these specific initiatives have actually been in improving workplace safety, and whether there is any empirical basis for providing an answer. We return to that question in the final section of this chapter.

Workplace Safety in Pennsylvania: Performance Data and Comparisons

There are several different data sources that can be used to examine trends in occupational injury and illness rates within Pennsylvania and comparable states. Within the commonwealth, BWC maintains records of all "first reports" of workplace injuries, which employers are required to submit in connection with any workplace incident involving a worker's fatality, permanent impairment, or loss of work time beyond the day or shift of occurrence (DLI, 2007b). Data elements available from the first reports include information on the employer's industry, the nature and cause of the worker's injury, age and gender of the injured worker, the part of the body affected by the injury, and the county within Pennsylvania where the injury took place. Summary statistics based on aggregated occupational injury and illness data are published annually by the Claims Management Division within BWC (BWC Claims Management Division, 2004, 2005, 2006).

For the most serious injuries and illnesses, the U.S. Bureau of Labor Statistics (BLS) maintains its own database of all traumatic workplace fatalities in the United States, called the Census of Fatal Occupational Injuries (CFOI). CFOI data are derived both from mandatory reporting of fatalities and from additional data sources, and these data are available online through BLS, from 1992 through the present (Bureau of Labor Statistics, 2008). In addition to CFOI, BLS also maintains an annual Survey of Occupational Injuries and Illnesses (SOII), which surveys approximately 175,000 employers each year to determine industry-specific injury rates. Recordable cases for this BLS survey differ somewhat from the cases that are included on the Pennsylvania first reports. Note that all but eight states have requested that the BLS increase the size of its survey sample within their own boundaries, in order to obtain state-specific injury rate estimates from the BLS survey. Unfortunately, Pennsylvania is one of the eight states that have not made this request. Consequently, it is more difficult to compare Pennsylvania's rates of industrial injury to those of other states and nationally. Finally, complementary data on workplace injury rates are also collected by OSHA through the "OSHA Data Initiative" (ODI), which targets particular groups of employers in different years to calculate lost workday injury rates for those sets of employers.

By combining BWC's historical data on the number of annual injuries in Pennsylvania with BLS data on the total number of employees in Pennsylvania in December of each year (shown in Table 3.1), we find that state injury rates have decreased from about 30 per 1,000 workers in 1980 to between 15 and 18 per 1,000 workers between 1996 and 2005. The degree to which this reduction is due to safety policies that were specifically introduced in Pennsylvania during the mid-1990s has not been established. The observed decrease in the injury rate

Table 3.1
Recent History of Pennsylvania Injury Rates

Year	Reported Injuries[a]	Employment[b]	Injury Rate (per 1,000)
1980	147,466	5,008,990	29.4
1990	158,030	5,475,313	28.9
1995	118,313	5,571,622	21.2
1996	102,132	5,735,777	17.8
1997	88,451	5,815,707	15.2
1998	85,783	5,790,559	14.8
1999	82,676	5,814,201	14.2
2000	80,133	5,854,749	13.7
2001	90,405	5,868,832	15.4
2002	95,206	5,830,483	16.3
2003	99,161	5,852,288	16.9
2004	93,566	5,938,829	15.8
2005	102,259	5,976,674	17.1

[a] According to BWC Claims Management Division (2006). DLI-reported injury rates are based on data reported to the Bureau of Workers' Compensation. Certain categories of labor, such as federal employees, maritime workers, and self-employed persons, are not included in BWC reporting requirements.

[b] According to BLS, Local Area Unemployment Statistics for December of each year.

may also be due, at least in part, to industry shifts over the same time period, as manufacturing decreased from employing more than 20 percent to less than 15 percent of the labor force, while the services industry increased from 25 percent to 33 percent of the labor force—a gradual shift toward occupation in less dangerous employment settings, following the decline of the commonwealth's steel industry (Bureau of Economic Analysis, 2007; Latzko, 2001). If the industry mix in Pennsylvania continues to move toward industries with fewer safety hazards, it is likely that the historical decline in injury/illness rates may continue into the future, even without additional policy changes.

More detailed statistics compiled by BWC indicate that the total number of injuries and illnesses reported in Pennsylvania has been fairly consistent over the last five years, albeit with a relatively low number in the 2004–2005 fiscal year and a relatively high number in the 2005–2006 fiscal year (DLI, 2007b). During the same period, the proportion of reported occupational injuries and illnesses that were fatal has remained between 1.1 and 1.5 per 1,000, a rate that has been roughly stable in this range since declining in the early 1990s. The highest raw numbers of occupational injuries over the past three years were reported in the industrial groups of "Trade, Transportation, and Utilities," "Manufacturing," and "Educational and Health Services," while the highest rates of injury were found in the "Natural Resources and Mining" group (51 per 1,000 workers), the "Construction" group (37 per 1,000 workers), the "Manufacturing" group (26 per 1,000 workers), and the "Trade, Transportation, and Utilities" group (20 per 1,000 workers) (BWC Claims Management Division, 2006). Similar to national data, strains and sprains account for 43 percent of all injuries in Pennsylvania, and overexertion is the leading type of accident or exposure at 31 percent. The majority of reported occupational injuries affected the upper or lower extremities (32 percent and 23 percent, respectively), with an additional 24 percent affecting the trunk. BWC provides further aggregate statistics, useful to insurers, safety professionals, employers, and workers in each industry, describing the breakdowns in types of injury, parts of body affected, and causes of injury within each major industry group (BWC Claims Management Division, 2006). While these Pennsylvania statistics may help point toward industries and types of accidents that create the greatest volume of injuries or where safety is a greater issue, they do not directly shed light on how Pennsylvania compares with other states on workplace safety, or on how effective instituted safety policies in the commonwealth have been.

As described above, BLS does not generate nonfatal injury rates for Pennsylvania from the SOII. And the information that is collected by BWC on injury rates is not directly comparable to the SOII data for other states. An alternative we consider here is to make use of the comparative information contained in the OSHA Data Initiative.[5] ODI data are obtained by OSHA from selected types of employers in different years. While the ODI sample does not provide a representative picture of all industries, the industries targeted in any given year are the same in all states, suggesting that the injury rates are likely to be comparable across states.[6] Table 3.2 presents results from ongoing research at the RAND Center for Health and Safety in the Workplace that uses the ODI data pooled across years 1995 through 2002 to calculate lost workday injury rates in several industry categories for Pennsylvania, eight other nearby states, and nationally. The industry categories shown (using two-digit Standard Industry Classification codes [SICs]) are those that are large enough such that there were at least 100 observations in the ODI data set for Pennsylvania. Among these industries, Pennsylvania injury rates were higher than the national rates for 23 of the 28 industries and were above the nine-state median of nearby states for 27 of the 28 industries. This set of industries is mostly contained within the manufacturing industrial group, which employs approximately 15 percent of the Pennsylvania workforce, with some additional industries in the retail and wholesale trade group, which covers another 20 percent of the commonwealth's workforce. Thus, while this method does not allow us to consider all major industry groups, the results for this subset suggest that Pennsylvania has occupational injury rates that are fairly high relative to national or regional rates, although almost always within the range of rates observed in local states.

For comparisons of occupational fatalities, we used the BLS Census of Fatal Occupational Injuries, which gathers data on acute events (not, for example, deaths due to illnesses from long exposures). We compared death rates per 100,000 workers for each of the major sectors in each state (manufacturing, construction, trade, etc.). Because the BLS does not publish data when the number of deaths in a category is three or fewer, we restricted the comparison to other states that were large enough to have rates presented for each sector. We chose to look at the ten most populous states, then eliminated the southern states (Florida, Georgia, and Texas), which tend to have historically higher rates. We ended up comparing fatality rates in Pennsylvania with those in California, New York, Illinois, Michigan, Ohio, and New Jersey

---

[5]   Note, however, that research has suggested that both the SOII and the ODI substantially undercount workplace injuries and illnesses, missing more than 30 percent of the eligible incidents. See Rosenman et al. (2006). It is not known whether this undercount varies considerably across states.

[6]   The industries described here are broad classifications, so if the types of industry (or establishment sizes) within these classes vary across states, and the safety risks vary across these subclasses, then the rates may not be fully comparable across states.

Table 3.2
Median Lost Work Day Rates from 1995–2002

Industry	PA	NY	NJ	OH	MD	WV	MI	IL	IN	National
PA > 8 states										
Construction, specialty trades	4.6	4.0	3.7	3.3	4.4	2.4	4.2	4.4	3.3	4.2
Air Transportation	8.1	6.6	6.8	5.7	4.7	4.8	6.0	7.9	5.5	6.8
PA > 7 states										
General Contractors	4.2	2.7	1.0	2.5	1.8	4.9	3.3	3.6	3.5	3.0
PA > 6 states										
Manufacturing, food	7.1	5.7	4.6	6.1	5.8	8.7	8.1	5.9	6.6	6.3
Manufacturing, textile mill	4.8	2.3	2.6	6.7	4.4	3.0	7.1	2.3	4.5	3.3
Manufacturing, furniture	6.5	4.1	4.2	5.3	4.2	10.3	8.2	4.7	6.2	5.3
Manufacturing, paper	4.8	3.7	3.5	3.8	4.6	5.8	6.3	4.0	4.7	3.9
Manufacturing, chemicals	2.7	2.6	2.0	2.4	2.7	1.1	3.0	2.6	2.8	2.4
Motor freight transportation and warehousing	6.1	5.1	4.5	5.0	5.0	6.2	7.5	6.0	5.7	5.7
Wholesale trade, nondurable	7.4	5.9	6.0	5.4	6.0	6.6	10.4	6.7	7.7	6.8
Retail trade, building, hardware, garden	5.5	4.3	3.5	5.3	5.2	9.4	4.1	5.4	8.4	5.4
Health services	9.0	7.5	6.9	6.3	5.9	12.1	10.0	6.3	8.1	7.3
PA > 5 states										
Manufacturing, lumber	7.0	5.8	5.8	6.4	4.8	8.4	6.5	7.1	7.6	6.0
Manufacturing, printing/ publishing	2.4	1.0	1.8	1.7	2.1	2.7	3.4	2.3	3.3	2.3
Manufacturing, primary metal	7.0	7.8	4.8	6.9	6.2	6.9	9.3	6.9	8.0	6.8
Manufacturing, fabricated metal	6.0	4.4	3.6	5.4	5.0	7.5	7.9	4.7	7.0	5.5
Manufacturing, transportation equipment	6.4	4.1	3.6	6.2	5.3	6.5	6.7	5.9	6.4	5.5
Manufacturing, misc. industries	4.4	1.9	2.0	4.0	4.2	4.8	5.3	3.1	4.8	3.5
Electric, gas and sanitary services	8.6	7.5	6.6	8.1	5.0	10.9	8.8	6.9	10.2	7.4
Wholesale trade, durable goods	6.1	4.7	4.5	5.6	5.8	7.2	6.8	4.9	7.7	5.6
PA > 4 states										
Manufacturing, apparel	2.2	0.00	0.7	3.4	1.9	4.5	6.6	1.9	5.5	2.4
Manufacturing, petroleum refining	2.2	3.6	1.2	2.0	0.0	2.7	2.6	1.1	3.5	1.7
Manufacturing, rubber, misc. plastics	5.2	4.1	3.4	5.8	5.0	6.4	7.9	4.3	6.4	5.2
Manufacturing, stone, clay, glass, concrete	5.7	5.0	3.8	5.2	6.4	8.3	6.9	4.8	6.1	5.3
Manufacturing, machinery, computer	3.4	3.2	2.1	3.3	2.2	6.7	4.8	3.9	4.3	3.7
Manufacturing, electronics	2.4	1.8	1.5	3.0	1.0	3.6	4.6	2.4	5.0	2.4
Manufacturing, instruments	1.9	1.5	1.1	1.0	0.8	2.5	3.5	2.0	2.1	1.7
PA > 2 states										
Retail trade, general merchandise	3.5	4.0	3.4	3.6	3.1	6.5	5.7	3.8	5.4	4.2

NOTES: These figures are based on establishment data collected as part of the OSHA Data Initiative for the years 1995–2002. Industry categories are two-digit SICs, and those shown are the two-digit SIC sectors in which Pennsylvania had more than 100 observations. The rates are lost workday injuries per 100 full-time equivalent workers (i.e. per 2,000 hours per year). We use the median rate rather than the mean because the former is less affected by extreme values. In each row, Pennsylvania and the states with injury/illness rates higher than Pennsylvania are shaded.

(see Table 3.3). For the ten industry sectors, Pennsylvania had the highest rate among the seven states in four sectors, the second-highest rate in two, the third-highest in two, the fourth-highest in one, and the fifth-highest in one. Thus, in only one sector did Pennsylvania have a rate that was lower than the median, while in eight sectors its rate was higher than the median. None of the other six states had an average ranking as high as Pennsylvania's.

Safety Compliance and Policy Initiatives: Performance Data and Assessment

As described earlier, there are at least three major safety policy initiatives that have been implemented in Pennsylvania during the past 15 years: the Act 44 mandates concerning the provision of accident-prevention services by insurers (and employers who self-insure); the institution of insurance rate incentives for employers with DLI-certified safety committees; and the broader efforts to increase attention to workplace safety and access to safety resources, such as the governor's WorkSAFE PA initiative and BWC's efforts to provide accessible and high-quality safety resources and training to the employment community. These state-specific policy efforts are in addition to the federal OSHA system of safety standards, inspections, and enforcement. In Pennsylvania, there is some published empirical work on the take-up and impact of the safety committee certification program, and nationally there is published work on the effects of being cited with a violation in an OSHA inspection.

A brief report by the Pennsylvania Compensation Rating Bureau on the commonwealth's safety committee certification program, together with the BWC's annual reports, show that the program has seen a steady increase in participation since its inception, with approximately 300 employers having certified safety committees in 1994 and approximately 4,800 applying for certification or renewal of certification in the 2005/2006 fiscal year (Pennsylvania Compensation Rating Bureau, 2006; DLI, 2007b). The cumulative number of workplace safety committee certification renewals now totals more than 26,000, and the cumulative amount that those employers have saved through safety credits due to participation in the program is

Table 3.3
Pennsylvania's Ranking Among Selected States in Traumatic Occupational Death Rate

Sector	Pennsylvania's Rank[a]
Agriculture	4th
Construction	2nd
Manufacturing	3rd
Transportation and public utilities	1st
Trade	1st
Professional and business services	1st
Education and health services	3rd
Leisure and hospitality services	1st
Other services	5th
Public administration	2nd

[a] Where "1st" represents the highest death rate.

well in excess of $100 million (DLI, 2007b). While the growth in program participation certainly reflects positively on the safety committee certification initiative, the PCRB reports that less than 1 percent of eligible insurance risks (a somewhat higher number than the number of eligible employers, since some employers may have more than one insurance policy in a given year) had their premiums reduced due to BWC certification of a safety committee over the first ten years of the program (1994–2003). Those participating tend to be larger employers, and they cover 8 percent of the total workers' compensation premiums paid across all eligible employers in Pennsylvania (Pennsylvania Compensation Rating Bureau, 2006).

The PCRB study does provide some evidence that the safety committee program in Pennsylvania may be having the desired effect of improving workplace safety at participating firms. In particular, the PCRB report compared the actual annual losses that participating and non-participating firms experienced with the standard premiums actually paid by each set of firms (Pennsylvania Compensation Rating Bureau, 2006). Because those premiums include adjustments based on experience ratings, they can be viewed as controlling for the history of prior losses at the firms, and they thus provide a measure of predicted losses in the future. Importantly, the PCRB report found that the ratio of actual losses to these "predicted losses" was lower for the participants in the commonwealth's safety committee program than for nonparticipants, a result that suggests improved safety performance, and reduced costs associated with injuries, at the participating firms (Pennsylvania Compensation Rating Bureau, 2006). This finding is promising, although further analyses are needed to rule out other possible explanations for it. For example, if participating firms tended to apply for certification in response to unusually poor recent safety performance, the improvements that they subsequently experienced may simply reflect a return to more typical levels of safety performance.

Results on the take-up of the commonwealth's safety committee program, on the other hand, are clear: The numbers of participating firms are low but increasing. At present, data are not available to assess the extent to which participating employers already had operating safety committees prior to their certification by the commonwealth, or the extent to which employers have safety committees of some form but choose not to participate in the state certification process.

With regard to the effects of OSHA safety standards and enforcement, research has shown that employers who have been fined for violations in the course of an OSHA inspection experience subsequent declines in their injury/illness rates, although the substantial declines seen in the early 1980s were much reduced by the late 1990s (Gray and Mendeloff, 2002; Mendeloff and Gray, 2005). The same studies also found that the rates of many different types of injuries were reduced, not just those that are specifically prevented by OSHA inspections or that were related to the particular standards cited. Related research has shown that OSHA health inspections have a significant impact on the regulatory compliance of firms that are inspected and that the threat of OSHA inspections results in a surprising amount of compliance, given the low likelihood of an OSHA inspection for any individual firm (Gray and Jones, 1991; Weil, 1996). More importantly, these sorts of empirical findings with regard to OSHA inspections suggest that mandatory safety standards with enforcement are capable of having positive effects on regulatory compliance and injury rates, at least in the short term, for those employers who actually receive inspections.

Unfortunately, there are no data currently available to assess the specific effects on safety outcomes of Pennsylvania's state mandates for the provision of accident-prevention services by insurers or employers who self-insure. Also yet to be systematically investigated are the effects on outcomes of the various state and DLI efforts to increase safety awareness and provide easier access to safety resources to employers. Given the paucity of evaluative data pertaining to these programs, an obvious priority for future reform would be to gather such data and to begin assessing the effects of the different initiatives.

Discussion and Policy Implications

Pennsylvania has been home to a variety of workplace safety initiatives, programs, and requirements over the course of the last 25 years. Some of those safety programs and requirements have been initiated through the Pennsylvania workers' compensation system and state law, while others have flowed through federal OSHA requirements or through nongovernmental organizations and partnerships. Against the backdrop of all this activity, Pennsylvania's actual safety performance, in terms of rates of occupational injuries, improved substantially between 1980 and 2005 (as reflected by workers' compensation reporting statistics). Direct comparisons between Pennsylvania injury rates and those of other states are more difficult to undertake, however, in part because Pennsylvania does not fully participate in the BLS Survey of Occupational Injuries and Illnesses. The more limited federal data that are available through the ODI and CFOI mechanisms suggest that Pennsylvania may not be a particularly strong performer on safety outcomes, when compared with other states on corresponding measures of lost workday injuries and fatal injuries. Meanwhile, state-level data and assessments describing the impact of specific Pennsylvania workplace safety policies are largely nonexistent, with the exception of a limited PCRB study that has examined some of the effects of certified workplace safety committees.

From the governor's office to the annual reports produced by the BWC, it is nevertheless clear that Pennsylvania government stakeholders see safety as a key driver in workers' compensation and that they consider continued improvement in workplace safety a high priority. The policies already enacted by the commonwealth to address workplace safety focus on a range of informational, technical, and cost barriers to improved safety performance among employers and insurers. In some cases, safety policies in the commonwealth have taken the form of collaborative efforts to increase awareness and provide resources, as through the WorkSAFE PA initiative. These efforts are clearly aimed at addressing the informational and technical barriers to superior safety outcomes. At the other end of the spectrum, safety policies in Pennsylvania have also taken the form of legislated mandates for insurers and self-insured employers to establish accident-prevention services, subject to monitoring and enforcement by the commonwealth. Falling in between the legislative mandates and purely voluntary efforts to increase safety awareness and access to information are voluntary policy initiatives that focus on cost incentives, such as the commonwealth's safety committee certification program and the state's OSHA consultation program, which provides free advice to small firms.

In stakeholder interviews with employers and insurers, we heard several positive responses to the support offered by BWC to employers in establishing safety committees and providing safety training for workers, as well as shared sentiment that safety has been important in reducing the volume of workers' compensation claims. We also heard positive reactions from at least one person concerning the usefulness of state audits in connection with the required provision of accident-prevention services by self-insured employers; the person we spoke with on this point indicated particularly that state audits have provided useful information for identifying weaknesses in existing safety programs, as well as for suggesting specific ways to improve those programs.

One stakeholder expressed concern about the difficulty of reaching out to employers about workplace safety, since employers generally resist expanding their relationships with the agencies of state or local government. This interviewee suggested that new mandates are likely to be the only way to reach members of the employer community who view the safety resources created by the state with suspicion and avoid participation in any program that will increase the government's "meddling in their business." Many of the features of the commonwealth's current safety initiatives involve state-run trainings/workshops and government provision of technical support—programs for which employer participation is elective rather than mandated.

Certified safety committees were raised as a topic of conversation in several interviews with employers, insurers, and officials, who suggested that this program in particular may be a topic for further policy development. The employers and insurers we spoke with were generally aware that the program exists and that there are signs suggesting it can be effective, but that take-up of the program among employers remains low. One option suggested in our interviews for possible future reform would involve expanding the reach of safety committees by mandating their establishment for all firms that do not self-insure, perhaps excluding smaller businesses from this requirement.

Short of instituting this kind of mandatory reform, though, several points of consideration for policymakers seem clear. First, it makes sense to think of safety as a key element of workers' compensation policy, because other factors and costs being equal, reducing occupational injuries is always more desirable than compensating for them after they occur. Second, despite the fact that Pennsylvania already has an abundance of safety-oriented policies in place, there has been very little data gathering or formal assessment to show where, and to what extent, those policies have actually worked in achieving their aims. More and better performance data, together with formal programmatic evaluations on a prospective basis, could be helpful to policymakers in refining existing safety mandates and initiatives and deciding whether to institute new ones.

Finally, as a matter of systems architecture, we believe that making good information on safety performance available to the employer community should be a top priority for policymakers in Pennsylvania. In principle, one of the strongest arguments favoring workplace safety reforms is that they may serve to benefit not only the interests of workers, but those of employers as well (by reducing workers' compensation costs and other productivity, regulatory, and reputational costs associated with workplace injuries). But that principle only operates if (1) an employer can quantify the marginal advantages associated with superior safety performance and (2) those advantages accrue to the benefit of the employer's bottom line. Thus, an ideal set of occupational safety policies in the commonwealth should make any corresponding reductions in workers' compensation costs as transparent, salient, and remunerative as possible to employers, in order better to align their natural interest in collaborating with workers to improve safety.

CHAPTER FOUR
Medical Care

A crucial aspect of any workers' compensation system is a set of mechanisms and standards for providing medical care to injured workers. Medical care is important in redressing the direct, physical effects of injury (and of hazardous exposure) in the workplace, and one criterion for evaluating a workers' compensation system involves looking at claimants' access to, outcomes from, and satisfaction with medical care. Medical care is also important because of its collateral effects on the indemnity side of workers' compensation: Addressing injuries quickly and effectively and returning claimants to their jobs and to the workplace can diminish the demand for indemnity benefits.[1] Meanwhile, costs associated with medical care in the workers' compensation system, as with the costs of medical care more generally, have been rising significantly and steadily on a national basis. At least one commentator has observed that it will be challenging to stem growth in workers' compensation medical costs in the future, for many of the same reasons that make it difficult to stem the growth in costs associated with employer-based health care coverage (Victor, 2003).

This chapter offers a summary review of evidence from several major empirical studies that have examined the performance of workers' compensation medical care in Pennsylvania. It also touches on several relevant policy issues in the commonwealth, drawing in part on input from stakeholders. Note that the review offered by this chapter is not intended to be comprehensive. Previous empirical studies on workers' compensation medical care are voluminous in themselves, contain their own summaries, and include an abundance of performance measures describing many aspects of care. Likewise, some important elements of workers' compensation medical policy, most notably concerning the structure and comparative strengths of the medical fee schedule, are also deeply complicated and beyond the scope of this chapter to address fully. Instead, our aim here is simply to present a distillation of some major performance findings, to clarify that health care quality, access, and cost each represent important criteria for evaluating system performance, and to identify some of the key policy issues that may be focal to future calls for reform in Pennsylvania.

As alluded to in Chapter One (see pp. 3–4), medical care in the Pennsylvania workers' compensation system has already been the subject of legislative change, most notably in the context of Act 44 in 1993. That Act established the state's current fee schedule for workers' compensation medical care, as well as standards and requirements concerning utilization review. Other aspects of the current medical framework, including the 90-day requirement

---

[1] On a similar note, some of the other categories of employer costs connected with workplace injuries, such as productivity losses and reputational harm, might also be mitigated by quick and effective medical care that returns injured workers more rapidly to their pre-injury employment.

29

for seeing an in-panel provider and the commonwealth's review mechanism concerning disputed medical fees, were established in 1996. Consonant with the reality that workers' compensation medical costs continue to climb, relevant policies in the commonwealth remain in flux. As of June 2007, for example, BWC had pending a set of proposed regulations, which, if implemented, would enact significant changes to Pennsylvania's rules governing medical cost containment, particularly regarding utilization review.[2] Given the nature of the health care landscape and the likelihood that pressure to contain costs will not abate any time soon, some basic questions about the Pennsylvania system follow: How well is the system doing on a range of measures of outcome, access, quality, and cost? What kinds of interstate performance comparisons have been made, and what do they tell us? And what are some of the major aspects of Pennsylvania policy that invite consideration as possible targets for additional reform?

Medical Costs in Pennsylvania: Performance Data and Comparisons

In Chapter Two, we outlined general findings on patterns of workers' compensation benefits paid, and employer costs, in Pennsylvania. Those findings included some breakdowns that looked specifically at medical benefits paid and at the medical component of costs, with the results that (1) aggregate medical benefits paid in Pennsylvania, and in the nation as a whole, grew far more rapidly than did indemnity benefits paid during 2000–2004, (2) average medical costs per claim in Pennsylvania were significantly lower than the median value across a group of 13 WCRI comparison states, and (3) average medical payments per claim grew more slowly in Pennsylvania than across the comparison group states over the 1997–2002 time period.

Moving beyond these general findings, WCRI also published a much more extensive study looking at Pennsylvania medical costs and utilization patterns in detail (Eccleston, Wang, and Zhao, 2005b). Relevant analyses explored Pennsylvania costs for hospital (outpatient) providers versus nonhospital providers, and for several specific categories of medical services within each of those settings. Perhaps unsurprisingly, one of the more prominent findings was that Pennsylvania's medical payments per claim fell well below the median among comparison group states, both for payments to hospital-based providers and for payments to nonhospital-based providers (Eccleston, Wang, and Zhao, 2005b).[3] Follow-up analyses looked at indices of price and utilization (the two major components of medical costs) and found that, for nonhospital providers, Pennsylvania fell below the median among comparison group states on both indices. By contrast, for hospital-based (outpatient) providers, Pennsylvania had the lowest price index, but highest utilization index, among the comparison group states (Eccleston, Wang, and Zhao, 2005b). Among other things, these results suggest that utilization of outpatient services in the commonwealth (as compared with other states) skewed somewhat more toward hospital-based providers—potentially an important finding, since hospital-based providers also tended to be more costly than their nonhospital-based counterparts (Eccleston, Wang, and Zhao, 2005b). Additional analyses in the WCRI study looked more specifically at patterns in price and uti-

---

[2]   See 36 Pa. B. 2913 (Commonwealth of Pennsylvania, 2006a).

[3]   More specifically, these analyses looked at payments to outpatient providers for claims with more than seven days of lost time, arising between October 2001 and September 2002 and evaluated as of March 2003. As with the other WCRI and NASI studies, the findings reported here derive from a complicated set of data collection and statistical methods, the details of which are described in Eccleston, Wang, and Zhao (2005a, p. 70).

lization indices for different provider specialties (Eccleston, Wang, and Zhao, 2005b). In contrast to the general finding of lower medical payments per claim in Pennsylvania than in the comparison group states, physical medicine services[4] stood out for generating higher payments per claim in Pennsylvania than in the comparison group states, during the most recent available year of data: a finding that was driven by higher rates of utilization for physical medicine services in Pennsylvania (Eccleston, Wang, and Zhao, 2005b). Although these findings are consistent with the more general picture of relatively low medical costs per claim in Pennsylvania, they also demonstrate that Pennsylvania shows some idiosyncratic patterns in service utilization, which from a pure cost perspective might not be optimal.

Some of the most interesting results from the WCRI work involved looking at time trends in medical prices and utilization across different types of providers and service categories. For purposes of illustration, Table 4.1 shows average annual rates of growth in prices (over the period from 1997–2002) for several different categories of nonhospital services and suggests that those prices were growing somewhat more rapidly in Pennsylvania than they were elsewhere. Table 4.2 shows average annual growth rates in utilization for the same services and suggests a more varied picture, with utilization growing more slowly in Pennsylvania than it did across other states for some, but not all, categories of service. WCRI has generated time trends for payments, prices, and utilization across a much broader set of medical services and specialties (including, for example, looking at physician and chiropractor services, hospital inpatient services, etc.), and a full discussion of those time trends has already been offered elsewhere (Eccleston, Wang, and Zhao, 2005b). For current purposes, it suffices to note that (1) prices and utilization are the two basic components of medical costs and (2) across a range of outpatient services, increasing costs in Pennsylvania appear more often to have been associated with changes in prices rather than changes in utilization (Eccleston, Wang, and Zhao, 2005b). This is a result that seems to invite scrutiny of the medical fee schedule in Pennsylvania, which we discuss later in this chapter. More generally, a review of the WCRI trends on medical service prices and utilization can help to pinpoint the drivers of growth in medical costs, and such

Table 4.1
Price Indices, Illustrative Growth Rates, WCRI (1997–2002)

Provider Type	Average Pennsylvania Growth Rate (%)	Average Growth Rate, WCRI 12-State Median (%)	Is Pennsylvania's Growth Rate Greater or Less Than the Median?
Nonhospital Evaluation and Management Services	5.2	4.3	Greater
Nonhospital Major Radiology Services	4.3	3.9	Greater
Nonhospital Minor Radiology Services	4.0	1.0	Greater
Nonhospital Surgical Services	4.3	3.9	Greater
Nonhospital Physical Medicine Services	3.3	2.3	Greater

SOURCE: Abstracted from *The Anatomy of Workers' Compensation Medical Costs and Utilization in Pennsylvania, 5th Edition*, Cambridge, Mass.: Workers Compensation Research Institute, 2005.

---

[4] The category of "physical medical services" was broadly defined to include physical therapy, chiropractic services, and other similar types of care, all of them billed under CPT (Current Procedural Terminology) codes 97xxx and 98xxx.

Table 4.2
Utilization Indices, Illustrative Growth Rates, WCRI (1997–2002)

Provider Type	Average Pennsylvania Growth Rate (%)	Average Growth Rate, WCRI 12-State Median (%)	Is Pennsylvania's Growth Rate Greater or Less Than the Median?
Nonhospital Evaluation and Management Services	–0.9	0.7	Less
Nonhospital Major Radiology Services	1.1	1.1	Same
Nonhospital Minor Radiology Services	1.2	3.1	Less
Nonhospital Surgical Services	1.9	–0.3	Greater
Nonhospital Physical Medicine Services	3.7	6.5	Less

SOURCE: Abstracted from *The Anatomy of Workers' Compensation Medical Costs and Utilization in Pennsylvania, 5th Edition*, Cambridge, Mass.: Workers Compensation Research Institute, 2005.

a review might be useful in seeking to refine the delivery of care while limiting cost growth. Again though, the broader context is that Pennsylvania appears to be well below the median among comparison group states, both in terms of average medical payments per claim across all claims and in terms of the growth rate in those medical payments over the 1997–2002 period (Eccleston, Wang, and Zhao, 2005b).

Quality of Care and Access to Care: Performance Data and Comparisons

Cost is by no means the only criterion on which to evaluate the delivery of health care. There are two other major performance dimensions in assessing any medical care delivery system. One of those dimensions is *quality*, or how good the medical care provided actually is. The other is *access*, or the degree to which patients can readily obtain care through the system. Each of these dimensions is complex in itself and poses significant challenges for performance measurement. Quality, for example, can be measured in terms of clinical outcomes, or in terms of clinical processes in care, or in terms of the structure and resources that support care (Donabedian, 1980, 1982). Ideally, one would want to be able to assess all of these aspects of health care quality, in the context of the workers' compensation system (Nuckols, 2007). In practice, however, available data for Pennsylvania are quite limited and are largely based on previous surveys, which have simultaneously focused on both access issues and quality in clinical outcomes. In the review that follows, we will briefly summarize major performance findings from the empirical survey data on Pennsylvania.

At the outset, it is important to recognize that concerns about the quality of workers' compensation medical care, and about workers' access to that care, are equally important to considerations of cost. This is so for two reasons. First, quality medical care is a fundamental part of the bargain between employers and employees that the workers' compensation system represents. Second, the net costs to employers associated with effective care may often be less than the net costs associated with ineffective care, particularly to the extent that good medical care can reduce employee time spent away from work (and the corresponding demand for indemnity benefits, reduction in employer economic productivity, etc.). A number of medical policy initiatives in the Pennsylvania system, such as the 90-day requirement for seeking care through an employer-designated provider panel, were primarily aimed at affecting costs of care but may also have had impact on health care quality, access, or both. Pursuant to a legislative mandate going back to Act 44, the Pennsylvania Department of Labor and Industry has for many years conducted an annual survey study investigating issues of access to care, and of worker outcomes, in the Pennsylvania system.[5] Overview summaries of results from recent years of the survey have been published and made available online; they include both descriptive statistics and analytical findings on access and quality of outcomes (DLI, 2003, 2004, 2005, 2006a).

Quality of Care

Pennsylvania's survey of injured workers includes questions addressing two major aspects of quality in outcomes: patient satisfaction and timeliness of return to work. With regard to satisfaction, approximately 83 percent of survey respondents indicated that they were either "satisfied" or "very satisfied" with the medical care they had received—a stable result during the three most recent years in which the survey was fielded (2003–2005) (DLI, 2006a). Similarly, approximately 82 percent of respondents indicated that the care they received through workers' compensation was at least as good as the care received through other types of medical coverage—again, a result that was stable over the three most recent years of the survey (DLI, 2006a). Finally, with regard to timeliness of return to work, survey respondents reported losing an average of 51 days from work due to their injuries in the 2005 survey, 48 days in the 2004 survey, and 52 days in the 2003 survey. Between 92 percent and 93 percent of respondents reported that they ultimately returned to work without subsequent re-injury, over the same three-year period (DLI, 2006a). Taken together, these results suggest that a majority of surveyed recipients of workers' compensation health care in Pennsylvania have reported being satisfied with their care and ultimately successful in their efforts to return to work. Note, however, that these results address only a very limited aspect of health care quality, and include neither detailed clinical outcome measures nor clinical process measures.

The quality results from the Pennsylvania surveys are interesting, and they suggest that many of the claimants in the Pennsylvania system have had reasonably positive experiences with their medical care. The findings are qualified, however, by the fact that response rates on the annual surveys have been low (around 20 percent) and that nonresponse has been associated with several demographic characteristics in the underlying population, including age and gender (DLI, 2005, 2006a). More important, the Pennsylvania surveys do not by themselves provide a basis for comparing Pennsylvania performance to other states, in regard to measures of either health care quality or access. However, WCRI conducted its own independent survey study of claimants who received medical benefits in four states (Pennsylvania, California, Massachusetts, and Texas) during 1998 and 1999 (Victor, Barth, and Liu, 2003). The WCRI survey included a number of health care quality measures pertaining to return-to-work outcomes (e.g., speed, sustainability, percentage of respondents not returning to work), as well as to workers' satisfaction with care provided. The WCRI survey also included several measures pertaining to access to care (e.g., timeliness of initial provider visits, problems getting needed services, problems getting to see desired providers).

---

[5]   Limited methodological details regarding the most recent annual surveys, and particularly the sampling and nonresponse characteristics of the respondents, are provided in DLI (2006a, p. 17).

Quality results from the WCRI survey showed that workers in Massachusetts and Pennsylvania reported generally better outcomes of care than did their counterparts in California and Texas—notwithstanding the fact that Massachusetts and Pennsylvania had lower medical payments per claim, and lower rates of utilization, than did the other two states. Pennsylvania ranked first (or tied for first) among the four states on several quality outcome measures relating to return to work, including speed of return to work, duration of first return to work, and the percentage of respondents who felt that they had not returned to work too soon. Pennsylvania ranked second among the four states across a number of quality measures relating to satisfaction with health care received, including percentages of respondents reporting either strong satisfaction or strong dissatisfaction with their overall care (Victor, Barth, and Liu, 2003). Although these findings are somewhat dated and limited to only four states, they at least suggest that Pennsylvania may compare reasonably well with other states on available survey measures of quality outcomes.[6]

Access to Care

Both the Pennsylvania and WCRI surveys also included questions to evaluate workers' *access* to care through the workers' compensation system. The Pennsylvania surveys included an item to assess whether injured workers were able to see a medical provider within 48 hours of experiencing a workplace injury. Between 85 and 90 percent of survey respondents indicated that they were indeed seen by a doctor within 48 hours (in each of the survey years from 2003–2005) (DLI, 2006a). The Pennsylvania surveys also collected data on waiting periods associated with appointments for different types of specialists; the results indicate that delays are most common in appointments with neurologists and neurosurgeons (DLI, 2006a).

Access to care issues were also addressed through interstate comparisons in the WCRI survey, drawing on several different measures, including respondents' satisfaction with the timeliness of their initial provider visits and the frequency of encountering "big problems" in obtaining desired medical services. Pennsylvania ranked second among the four states (again, Massachusetts, Pennsylvania, California, and Texas) across several of these related access-to-care measures (Victor, Barth, and Liu, 2003). Again, we could imagine a range of other possible empirical measures that might provide more detailed information about access to care in the Pennsylvania system (e.g., the availability of specialists, delays or challenges associated with particular clinical procedures, frequency of utilization review challenges or denials of requested services). Nevertheless, the available survey data on access do suggest that Pennsylvania compares reasonably well with several peer states.

Beyond the general Pennsylvania survey findings on quality outcomes and access to care, the annual Pennsylvania survey has also been used to explore the association between quality outcomes, access measures, and some specific workers' compensation policies (e.g., promoting access to care through provider panels). We describe a few pertinent results below, in addressing related policy issues. On a different point, we note that the annual Pennsylvania survey has also included a module for surveying insurers and providers (DLI, 2006a). Although the commonwealth has not published details of sampling and methods for this part of its annual

---

[6]   After work on this report was completed, WCRI published a new survey study comparing workers' compensation medical care outcomes, costs, and utilization patterns across nine states. See Belton, Victor, and Liu (2007). Findings from this survey study reportedly place Pennsylvania above the median among the nine comparison states in terms of the value of medical care provided (i.e., relatively low costs together with superior outcomes).

survey, the findings are nevertheless relevant to shifting patterns in access to care. In particular, the surveys have been used to compute "voluntary attrition" rates among physicians who saw workers' compensation patients, based on the physicians' reports of having reduced or terminated their workers' compensation caseloads. The rate of voluntary attrition has reportedly fluctuated between 11 and 27 percent among surveyed providers over the most recent three years (DLI, 2004, 2005, 2006a). These attritions have been interpreted as problematic in DLI's published summary reports, although the attritions may have been partly offset by an unspecified number of new physicians who enter into delivering workers' compensation care each year. Results from both the provider and insurer surveys suggest that there have been particular problems in maintaining pools of available providers in some medical specialties such as orthopedic surgery, neurosurgery, and neurology (DLI, 2006a).

Data Limitations

Ultimately, the available survey data on health care quality and access within the Pennsylvania system may be most striking for their limited coverage, in relation to the broader performance domains that they seek to address. As one recent reviewer has noted, quality measurement in workers' compensation health care has lagged behind similar efforts within the wider U.S. health care system (Nuckols, 2007). Ideally, one would want to be able to measure quality through a range of detailed clinical outcomes and also through process indicators (that, for example, are designed to capture providers' compliance with published clinical practice guidelines). In practice, this kind of measurement is still in early development with regard to workers' compensation medical care (Nuckols, 2007). We are left to speculate whether research findings suggesting poor quality performance in general health care across the United States, together with systematic under-use of appropriate medical services, would apply similarly in the workers' compensation context (McGlynn et al., 2003; Nuckols, 2007). Developing better measurement resources and data to address this question should be a high priority for policymakers and researchers alike.

Policies in Workers' Compensation Medical Care

In light of concerns about rising health care costs in workers' compensation, Pennsylvania instituted a number of changes in the 1990s. Those reforms included the current medical fee schedule; panel requirements for workers seeking to obtain care (during the first 90 days following injury); standards and procedures for utilization review; and a mechanism for resolving disputes between providers and insurers over medical fees. According to one stakeholder in the insurance community with whom we spoke, the initial set of legislative reforms in 1993 had a pronounced effect in helping to bring down medical cost growth in the commonwealth. By implication, the reforms probably contributed to the WCRI empirical results on medical costs in Pennsylvania that we described earlier, as well as to the general finding that Pennsylvania has lower costs per claim than do a number of other states on several measures of medical payments. Nevertheless, the most recent NASI data on medical payments in Pennsylvania suggest that those payments are continuing to rise and that they are doing so at a more rapid rate than indemnity payments. Given the likelihood of continuing growth in medical costs, future calls for additional policy reform and medical cost containment seem probable. In the context of this environment, we summarize here some of the major avenues for reform in medical policies, both to review the impact of what has already been tried in Pennsylvania and to discuss what might be tried in the future.

Networks and Panel Access

One of the major policy changes instituted during the last 20 years has been to expand the length of time during which workers are required to seek treatment through an employer-designated provider panel. Pennsylvania law does not require that employers establish such provider panels, but if they do, workers then have the obligation to seek care through the panels for the first 90 days following workplace injury. Several of the stakeholders with whom we spoke specifically mentioned provider panels as having had a positive effect in Pennsylvania, either in controlling costs or in helping to give workers easier access to multiple medical providers who accept workers' compensation cases.[7] These anecdotal accounts are consistent with empirical findings on the effect of panels. In the most recent year of the Pennsylvania DLI study, 79 percent of workers surveyed reported having access to provider panels through their employers (DLI, 2006a). The DLI survey also found that access to care through a panel was associated with increasing levels of satisfaction with care over the 2000–2004 interval (DLI, 2005) and, moreover, that panel access in 2005, when compared with lack of panel access, was associated with higher levels of satisfaction and superior outcomes across several self-reported survey measures (DLI, 2006a). On a complementary note, a literature review on provider networks in workers' compensation suggested, for several states other than Pennsylvania, an association between the use of networks and reductions in medical costs per claim (Victor, 2003). Taken together, Pennsylvania data and anecdotal accounts suggest that provider panels have become a primary avenue for obtaining medical treatment through workers' compensation and that panels have been associated with some beneficial effects on health care quality (outcomes) and on access to care in the commonwealth.

To the extent that provider panels in Pennsylvania can simultaneously generate reduced costs and superior outcomes, they clearly represent a win-win policy device for workers and employers. To the best of our knowledge, however, the cost impact of panels in Pennsylvania has not yet been evaluated empirically, and even the clinical impact of panels has been subject only to limited and retrospective scrutiny. Better data and analysis on these points could be useful to policymakers in deciding what changes, if any, should be made to current panel requirements. In the meantime, we see several potential options for building on the existing framework for panels in the commonwealth. One stakeholder suggested to us that the current 90-day requirement for seeking treatment through a panel should be expanded to 180 days, to provide better management of care for serious injuries while reducing the frequency of defections by workers to more costly nonpanel medical providers. Another option for reform could involve increasing the availability and penetration of panels throughout Pennsylvania, such as by enacting new incentives or mandates for employers to adopt panels for their workers. In either case, we would ideally want to gauge the effects of any policy change, in order to determine whether new initiatives are successful at achieving their desired aims. One method for doing this involves pilot studies, in which proposed reforms are instituted on a trial basis

---

[7]   Provider panels can theoretically have mixed effects on workers' access to medical care. On one hand, panels, by definition, restrict access to a specific list of medical providers. On the other hand, the existence of an employer-designated panel may sometimes make it easier for workers to identify and connect with providers, especially in otherwise underserved locations (e.g., rural areas).

in limited regions, with formal assessment and comparison with control regions. Regardless, any future policy initiatives to modify panel requirements should be accompanied by efforts to gather more information about panels, how they are being implemented, and what kinds of effects they have on injured workers and on medical costs.

Fee Schedule

A prominent theme that emerges in any policy discussion about the medical aspects of the Pennsylvania workers' compensation system involves the commonwealth's medical fee schedule. As implemented by Act 44 in 1993, that fee schedule was originally based on Medicare, with subsequent annual adjustments tied to the growth in Pennsylvania's statewide average weekly wage rate. In the intervening years, though, the underlying Medicare fee structure has shifted in ways not reflected by Pennsylvania (Eccleston and Zhao, 2004), and the growing disparity between Pennsylvania's fee schedule and Medicare has given rise to calls for reform. One complaint about the Pennsylvania fee schedule that we heard in several stakeholder interviews is that many of its details are complex and difficult to process—a viewpoint that echoed the Legislative Budget and Finance Committee's description of the administrative challenges associated with implementing a fee schedule derived from Medicare circa 1994 (LBFC, 2005). On a different point, another stakeholder suggested to us that the current Pennsylvania fee schedule overcompensates some categories of specialists while undercompensating primary care physicians, in a manner that may create perverse incentives for treatment by more expensive providers. If true, this would imply that the fee schedule may be contributing to undesirable patterns in both medical prices and utilization, in ways not consistent with the schedule's basic aim of containing costs.

There have been a number of attempts to look empirically at recent years of the Pennsylvania medical fee schedule and to compare it with corresponding rates under Medicare (or under other insurance-based fee schedules within the commonwealth). The annual DLI survey study notably includes a module that compares Pennsylvania fees with those of Medicare for approximately 55 CPT codes each year (DLI, 2003, 2004, 2005, 2006a). The published results from (and methods behind) these fee comparisons are not well described, but the most recent DLI study indicated that workers' compensation fees averaged 128 percent those of Medicare across 54 sampled CPT codes in 2005. At the same time, though, the DLI study also found that Pennsylvania fees were actually below those of Medicare for 20 of the 54 sampled procedures (DLI, 2006a). A more detailed investigation of the Pennsylvania fee schedule was undertaken by WCRI in 2004. That study found that the Pennsylvania fee schedule had resulted in surgical and radiological procedures being much more highly compensated than under Medicare (at premiums ranging from 28 to 73 percent, by region), while physical and general medicine procedures were comparatively undercompensated (at premiums above Medicare ranging from 2 to 16 percent) (Eccleston and Zhao, 2004). The WCRI study also found that evaluation and management services, notably including physician office visits and consultations, were actually compensated at rates 4 to 7 percent *below* those of Medicare across much of Pennsylvania (Eccleston and Zhao, 2004).

Continuing comparisons between the Pennsylvania fee schedule and Medicare can offer some useful insights about the evolution of the former, particularly given that the Pennsylvania fee schedule was originally based on the Medicare framework from many years ago. Nevertheless, one interesting comment that we heard from a stakeholder was that there is no fundamental reason why Pennsylvania's updated fee schedule *should* match closely with contemporary

Medicare, since workers' compensation and Medicare deal with qualitatively different groups of beneficiaries and medical problems. Several interviewees also commented that the reality of medical fees under workers' compensation is frequently determined by managed care contracts, at rates that may be significantly discounted from the commonwealth's schedule. These kinds of observations underline the need for better empirical information, not only about the fee schedule itself, but also about the medical fees actually paid in Pennsylvania and how those fees vary by categories of service. In the meantime, proposals to shift Pennsylvania to a new fee schedule based on current Medicare practices would inevitably involve (1) a lot of highly technical details in the transition and (2) significant groups of winners and losers within the provider community. We note that a similar proposed transition in California was the subject of an extensive study that examined in detail the potential impact of revisions to the fee schedule, and how best to implement them (Wynn, 2003). Given that the pressure to contain medical costs in workers' compensation will likely continue for the foreseeable future, it may make sense to undertake a similar study for the Pennsylvania system, as a predicate to any proposal for major revision to the fee schedule designed to more aggressively contain costs.

Utilization Review and Disputes over Medical Billing

Apart from mechanisms such as the Pennsylvania fee schedule and provider panels, there are a number of other policy levers for controlling medical costs within the workers' compensation system. An important mechanism that was formally instituted in Pennsylvania by Act 44 is utilization review (UR). Under the provisions of the statute, utilization review in connection with disputed medical care can be requested by workers, employers, or insurers and must be conducted by an organization specifically authorized by the commonwealth for that purpose. Where disputes over the reasonableness or necessity of care persist despite findings from UR, the parties to the dispute can petition for review by a workers' compensation judge. In the context of health care more generally, UR is a device for containing costs by establishing independent oversight of the appropriateness of care, with the possibility for denial of requested services where these appear unreasonable to the reviewer; not surprisingly, this is a practice that sometimes gives rise to controversial results. In several conversations with Pennsylvania workers' compensation physicians, though, we were told that requests for UR had occurred only rarely in their experience and that these were not a major factor in their practice of occupational medicine. Published data on UR outcomes in Pennsylvania is scant, other than that approximately 7,000 requests for UR have occurred in each of the two most recent years, with about 1,800 cases per year ultimately resulting in petitions for judicial review of contested UR decisions (DLI, 2006b, 2007b).

Notwithstanding the above, it is nevertheless a timely point at which to consider the impact of UR, because as of 2007, the Bureau of Workers' Compensation had proposed some significant revisions to the regulations that implement the UR statute.[8] The proposed regulations go into much greater detail than before about how UR is supposed to work and what the corresponding rights and duties of the parties (and in particular, of employers and insurers) actually are. Presumably, the proposed regulatory changes on UR will help to clarify existing ambiguities in the system. Less clear is whether any of the proposed changes might have the effect of making UR more rigorous as a cost-containment device, such as by clarifying or

8   See 36 Pa. B. 2913 (Commonwealth of Pennsylvania, 2006a).

expanding the rights of insurers to seek UR on a prospective (pre-approval) basis or to request UR in advance in connection with all treatment decisions relating to a given worker. In any event, the fact that proposed regulations are currently under review suggests that there is an interest among stakeholders in refining the performance of the existing system: Assuming that the new regulations are adopted, it will be important to look at Pennsylvania's utilization review processes going forward and to examine the influence of the new rules on requests for review, on disputes, and ultimately on costs and impact on quality of care.

Although UR did not come up as a major issue in any of our interviews with stakeholders, one workers' compensation physician did comment to us on another dimension of medical cost-containment that had reportedly become problematic. That respondent described an increasing frequency of disputes between Pennsylvania providers and insurers over medical fees. In particular, the respondent suggested that some insurers had become aggressive in "down-coding" medical claims, thereby reducing payments while shifting the onus to providers to challenge the down-coding on a case-by-case basis.[9] Interestingly, there is some published evidence showing that formal conflicts between providers and insurers over medical fees are on the rise in Pennsylvania: According to BWC, the rate of formal medical fee reviews increased by 32 percent between FY 2003/2004 and FY 2004/2005 (to 18,935), and then again by 52 percent between FY 2004/2005 and FY 2005/2006 (to 28,194) (DLI, 2006b, 2007b). Although these statistics show that more and more disputes over payment are being brought to the state for formal review by providers, we note that the statistics do not, by themselves, reflect evidence of insurer down-coding. In particular, some of these disputes may well have focused on other sorts of payment issues (e.g., timeliness), and even for those disputes that did focus on coding in claims payment, it is also possible that many of them may have reflected legitimate problems with providers' billing or documentation rather than with insurers' re-coding practices. In sum, this is an issue that cannot be resolved directly through currently published summary statistics. Nevertheless, it is also an issue for which BWC may be able to offer more insight through its own review files, by looking at patterns in medical fee disputes and in who prevailed on the merits, over time. We believe that it makes sense for policymakers to track this issue going forward, because the rapid growth of fee disputes in recent years could indicate that a new systemic problem may be emerging.

Discussion and Policy Implications

Medical care in the Pennsylvania workers' compensation system is likely to be critical as a driver of growth in system costs in the future. Several corresponding observations are worth making here. First, many of the basic challenges associated with delivering and financing health care apply regardless of the unique context of workers' compensation. More than one stakeholder observed to us that the "real" solution to problems posed by workers' compensation medical care would involve implementing universal, single-payer health coverage and, by implication, eliminating the distinction that currently exists between ordinary health benefits and workers' compensation health benefits. That kind of proposal is deeply speculative in terms of its details

---

[9] Similar claims about down-coding by medical insurers have become the focus of high-profile litigation outside the context of workers' compensation in Pennsylvania and have resulted in some large settlement payments to physicians. See, for example, Connolly, (2005) and Stark (2004).

and ultimate effects, but it does reflect the reality that many aspects of health care costs are being driven by forces outside the scope of workers' compensation *per se*. To the extent that broader trends toward rising costs in health care continue throughout the United States, Pennsylvania will be compelled to confront and manage those costs in the more limited context of its workers' compensation system, with the specific policy levers that are available there.

In this chapter, we focused on discussing several of those policy levers, including employer panels, the workers' compensation fee schedule, and utilization review. Obviously, these are not the only mechanisms in play in delivering workers' compensation medical care. Various other forms of case management, price regulation, clinical care guidelines, pay-for-performance, and/or utilization controls could also be applied to the system, some of them with the potential for far-reaching effects on cost, quality, and/or access to services. Nevertheless, the mechanisms discussed in this chapter stand out as major health care policies already implemented in Pennsylvania, any of which could be further modified in the future in pursuit of additional cost containment (or quality) goals. Therefore, we see these policies as a logical starting point for policymakers in evaluating the effects of Pennsylvania's current framework for delivering medical care in the workers' compensation system, as well as in considering possible avenues for future reform. We note that available performance data concerning the specific impact of specific medical policies in Pennsylvania (such as the fee schedule or the use of provider panels) are currently quite limited. A key element in any future policy changes should be to gather prospective data on their impact on health care services.

In the meantime, current information on the performance of workers' compensation medical care suggests that, on several measures related to costs, Pennsylvania's system appears to fall below the median values among a group of comparison states. The limited available data also suggest that Pennsylvania compares reasonably well to several other states on survey measures of quality outcomes and access. This said, the broadest trends in the performance data suggest that medical payments in workers' compensation are going up everywhere, at rates substantially in excess of those for growth in indemnity benefits. This pattern suggests that containment of medical costs may become an increasingly important priority for the workers' compensation system in Pennsylvania, as well as in many other states, in years to come.

Finally, we conclude by observing that the performance of the Pennsylvania system in delivering medical care cannot be evaluated solely in terms of cost; it also requires the assessment of access to care and of health care quality (the latter including, but not limited to, clinical outcome measures such as speed of return to work). The legislature recognized this back in 1993, when it first mandated that the Department of Labor and Industry perform an annual survey study focusing on workers' access to quality care. More detailed information on the quality of workers' compensation health care, particularly on an interstate basis, could be particularly useful to policymakers in trying to understand how well Pennsylvania's system is actually doing. Even more important, though, is the recognition that the balance between cost on one hand, and quality and access on the other, reflects a fundamental tension between competing interests in the system. By corollary, the best prospects for future reform may involve breaking that duality, and finding ways to simultaneously control workers' compensation costs while maintaining or improving health care access and quality.

CHAPTER FIVE

Dispute Resolution

Disputes over workers' compensation claims arise between workers and employers (and their insurers) when claims for benefits submitted by the former are rejected or challenged by the latter. Disputed claims can arise in connection with a number of different legal and medical issues, including entitlement to benefits and the putative workplace causation of an injury, disability status, and benefits following recovery from injury. When disputes over these sorts of issues arise in the Pennsylvania system, they are dealt with primarily by the workers' compensation judges in the Office of Adjudication. In effect, these workers' compensation judges provide a specialized justice mechanism for dealing with disputes over benefits, removed from the trial courts of general jurisdiction in Pennsylvania. The initial level of appeal in the workers' compensation system is also handled through a specialized mechanism, the Workers' Compensation Appeals Board. A unique set of procedural rules and substantive standards apply to cases that are brought (or appealed) within the workers' compensation framework. And as noted in Chapter One, a number of aspects of this system have been modified by legislative reforms in the past ten years, including trial scheduling requirements, compromise and release agreements, mediation, and supersedeas proceedings (i.e., proceedings to modify or terminate benefits).

It is a matter generally agreed upon that efficient, inexpensive, and equitable resolution of disputes is an important factor in the successfulness of workers' compensation in fulfilling its purpose. Yet the dispute resolution system in Pennsylvania has been the subject of some historical criticism, particularly so during the 1990s, when the system was described as being highly litigious and subject to greater-than-average litigation costs in comparison with other states (LBFC, 2005). Given that the system has undergone significant changes in more recent years, several questions about it now arise. How well does Pennsylvania currently perform on benchmarks related to efficiency and cost in dispute resolution, and what are the trends on such measures over recent years? Is there any basis for performance comparison with other states? And are there important aspects of performance not currently being captured by available data? An equally important set of questions arises about dispute resolution policies in Pennsylvania, the impact of recent targeted reforms, and the prospects and priorities for additional potential changes in the future. We address these questions of performance and policy, together with available evidence from published data, in the discussion that follows.

The Dispute Resolution System in Pennsylvania: Performance Data and Comparisons

The Office of Adjudication publishes summary data on the volume of cases passing through the Pennsylvania system (which has remained relatively stable in recent years) and on the speed with which the system processes workers' compensation cases. Figure 5.1 shows that the average time from filing of a review petition to decision in those cases fell from 9.3 months in 2002 to 8.0 months in 2005 (DLI, 2007b). The Office of Adjudication also reported that time lag from petition to decision had decreased from 11.5 months in 1998, a finding that suggests an improving trend in speed of resolution in recent years, with cases being resolved considerably more quickly now, on average, than they were at the end of the 1990s. Another measure of performance tracked by the state is the fraction of cases for which decisions are rendered within 90 days of the closing of a petition (i.e., after a hearing on the merits). Ninety-five percent of cases in 2004, and 97 percent of cases in 2005, met this 90-day criterion. Meanwhile, the backlog of pending cases fell from approximately 35,000 to 32,000 during the same interval (DLI, 2006b, 2007b). It is unclear whether these latter improvements reflect a more enduring trend toward efficiency within the system, because the state has only provided the most recent year of summary data on the pending caseload and 90-day compliance rates in each of its last two annual reports.

Comparing these sorts of Pennsylvania performance statistics to those of other states is problematic for several reasons, most importantly because there is no single repository for this kind of dispute resolution data across states and because, even to the extent that data is available, the standards and processes for workers' compensation litigation vary across the states. Notably, some states do publish annual reports with summary statistics describing workers'

Figure 5.1
Average Time to Hear and Decide Cases in Pennsylvania

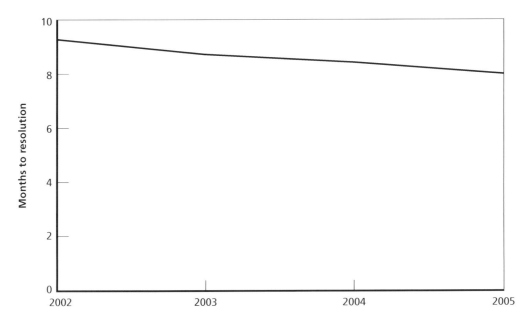

SOURCE: Abstracted from statistics in DLI (2007b).
RAND OP216-5.1

compensation litigation (e.g., Pennsylvania, New York, Illinois, Oregon), while others apparently do not (e.g., New Jersey, Indiana, Ohio, West Virginia). But even for those states that do, there is little harmony in the specific types of performance data that are reported. Thus, for example, New York does not provide statistics on average time to hear and decide cases but does describe the volume of cases passing through its system and the number of cases that were resolved through an initial pre-hearing conference process (New York State Workers' Compensation Board, 2005). The only other states for which we were able to obtain report data that describes speed in resolving cases were Illinois and Oregon. Illinois publishes statistics on the "turnaround time" from the original filing of a workers' compensation claim to the filing of a decision from the initial level of review (Illinois Workers' Compensation Commission, 2006), which unfortunately is not conceptually equivalent to Pennsylvania's "time to hear and resolve cases." Oregon, on the other hand, publishes summary statistics on the lag between initial hearing requests and the issuance of orders by its workers' compensation judges. In 2005, the median lag in Oregon was reportedly 146 days, or approximately five months (Oregon Department of Consumer and Business Services, 2006), as compared with Pennsylvania's eight months on a loosely analogous measure. We would caution that it is not at all clear how comparable the Pennsylvania and Oregon statistics truly are, but Oregon's shorter lag at least suggests that further improvement in Pennsylvania's speed in processing cases might be possible.

With regard to litigiousness and litigation expenses, WCRI has undertaken an extensive study on workers' compensation costs across a group of 13 states including Pennsylvania, notably incorporating specific observations on medical-legal expenses (i.e., in connection with disability assessments) and defense attorney involvement and costs in contested claims (Telles, Wang, and Tanabe, 2006b, 2006d).[1] Without recapping the most recent year of WCRI findings in detail, they are noteworthy for showing that Pennsylvania was at the median among the comparison group of states in terms of the frequency of defense attorney involvement (in claims with more than seven days of lost work time) and that Pennsylvania was only slightly above the median among the comparison states for average defense attorney costs per claim (Telles, Wang, and Tanabe, 2006b). Five-year time trends on the same WCRI measures of defense attorney involvement and costs suggest that Pennsylvania was roughly in line with median annual growth rates among the comparison states for both of these measures (Telles, Wang, and Tanabe, 2006d). By contrast, Pennsylvania had somewhat higher medical-legal expenses than did most of the WCRI comparison states, a finding that WCRI attributed in part to Pennsylvania's reliance on medical depositions, rather than reports, in workers' compensation proceedings (Telles, Wang, and Tanabe, 2006d). We return to that latter procedural issue in our discussion below.

Apart from costs and speed-of-processing measures, another potential dimension in gauging the performance of a dispute resolution system involves assessing the quality of the decisions that it reaches. That can be a difficult determination to make, however, since there is rarely an objective basis for classifying some decisions as "good" and others as "bad." Some states do report on the fraction of workers' compensation decisions at the trial court level that are appealed (Oregon Department of Consumer and Business Services, 2006) or that are reversed on appeal (Illinois Workers' Compensation Commission, 2006). These are imperfect measures of quality in adjudication, although lower rates of appeal and overturned decisions presumably

---

[1]   The WCRI findings described here are based on multistate descriptive statistics that were adjusted to control for states' industry mix, injury mix, and differential wage patterns. See discussion in Telles, Wang, and Tanabe (2006c, p. 68).

reflect better performance by trial courts than higher rates would. Regardless, Pennsylvania does not include either of these sorts of performance measures in its annual reports. During our interviews with Pennsylvania workers' compensation attorneys, one person suggested that it might be useful to generate a new measure of quality for judicial decisionmaking, such as asking both the plaintiff and defense counsel in each dispute to submit to the state anonymous ratings of judicial performance and of the legal complexity of the case in question. This kind of quality measure would go considerably beyond what any of the states we checked appear to be doing. In the absence of such methods, we observe that the available summary data on litigation costs and speed of dispute resolution in Pennsylvania present only a partial picture of the actual performance of the system in the commonwealth.

Policy Issues in Workers' Compensation Adjudication in Pennsylvania

One of the major focal points in recent efforts to reform the workers' compensation system has been on adjudication and dispute resolution mechanisms. This focus was reflected in both Act 57 (1996) and in Act 147 (2006), through the introduction (and revision) of compromise and release procedures, formal mediation processes, new standards in supersedeas proceedings, and the introduction of an increasingly rigorous set of professional standards within the workers' compensation judiciary (particularly at the WCAB level). A similar focus on litigation and dispute resolution was evident in the 2005 report of the Legislative Budget and Finance Committee, in which the authors noted that Pennsylvania had high legal costs associated with its workers' compensation system and included a number of recommendations for reducing those costs, such as implementing mandatory mediation, reducing serial hearings, and revising the statutory cap on plaintiff attorney fees to below 20 percent (LBFC, 2005). Although our own review of the most recent WCRI evidence on litigation costs suggests that Pennsylvania is not radically out of line with peer group states, we nevertheless recognize that continued improvement in resolving disputes has the potential to drive down employer and government costs even further. In the discussion that follows, we review several specific aspects of workers' compensation policy that have been targeted by past reforms, describe what has (or has not) been changed through legislation, and discuss implications for policy in the future.

With regard to litigation patterns in the Pennsylvania system more generally, we heard a number of relevant comments through our interviews with stakeholders (and particularly with workers' compensation lawyers). First, several people expressed agreement that the volume of litigation in Pennsylvania has diminished over the last five to ten years, perhaps most importantly because of increased workplace safety and a declining rate of industrial injuries. Second, despite the declining volume of litigated claims, stakeholders articulated a number of factors that continue to contribute to litigation within the system. These factors include poor communication and (putatively avoidable) misunderstandings between workers and employers over medical-only claims; mass media coverage about high-value tort settlements that may inflate workers' perceptions of their own injuries; and "preemptive" filing of petitions to preserve workers' compensation rights against the statute of limitations, even where the immediate need for benefits may not be clear. Notwithstanding these factors, people on both sides of the bar suggested that the system, at present, is working reasonably well. Another person commented that continuing calls for reform are driven by the perception that there is still a delay in resolving cases, despite the fact that the system has gotten much faster and reduced its case backlog over the last ten years. All parties agreed that the system has undergone substantial changes since 1996 and that future prospects for reform need to be understood in terms of changes that have already been made.

Serial Hearings

One aspect of workers' compensation adjudication that has periodically been criticized in Pennsylvania is "serial-style" hearings. Current state law does not require workers' compensation judges to resolve their cases during a single hearing ("one-day-one-trial"), but instead allows judges flexibility in deciding how to use and structure hearings in support of deciding their cases. In practice, this means that judges can hold multiple preliminary hearings in a case to obtain evidence, and also that different judges may engage in different practices with regard to their use of hearings. One of the specific recommendations from the 2005 LBFC report was to curtail serial hearings in favor of a one-day-one-trial approach, in which parties would be encouraged (or perhaps required) to present an entire case before the judge in a single day (LBFC, 2005). In principle, this kind of approach can save time by reducing scheduling burdens associated with litigation, as well as by pressing counsel to conduct pre-trial preparations with maximal efficiency. Likewise in principle, the savings in time could also translate into a corresponding savings in administrative and litigation expenses.

Interestingly though, the input we obtained from stakeholder interviews on this question was unenthusiastic. Lawyers on both sides of the workers' compensation bar expressed skepticism about the putative savings that would result from the one-day-one-trial approach. One person suggested that any savings in time would only accrue to the court itself (and not to counsel) and that cases under one-day-one-trial might be less likely to settle, since each side would first want to hear the other's testimony: a self-defeating result if true. Another person suggested that to make a one-day-one-trial system effective, the system would need to implement formal discovery procedures akin to those in civil litigation: again, a result that was construed as being worse than the problem it was intended to solve. Some of these comments appear to recap points that were made previously in legislative hearings in September, 2005, both by attorneys and an official from the Department of Labor and Industry (Greenberg, 2005). Perhaps the definitive summary of arguments about the merits and drawbacks of the Pennsylvania serial hearing approach was offered by Torrey and Greenberg (2002). They noted that a number of counties in the commonwealth had already experimented with one-day-one-trial procedures and that, although many of the procedures had been implemented successfully, there was no evidence to show that they were faster, simpler, or fairer than the status quo. Torrey and Greenberg went on to suggest that the serial hearing approach offered a number of distinct advantages, such as promoting more flexible discovery; strengthening parties' sense of participation in, and being heard by, the justice system; and better accommodating Pennsylvania's status as a "wage-loss" state, in which a claimant's permanent disability status (and entitlement to benefits) remains dynamic and subject to renewed challenge over time.

In light of the above, it is perhaps not surprising that a uniform, one-day-one-trial mechanism has not been implemented in any of the three major rounds of Pennsylvania legislative reform during the past 15 years. On the other hand, Act 147 did take a step in a related direction in 2006, by instituting mandatory trial scheduling for workers' compensation proceedings. That mandate requires judges to establish a full litigation schedule in the first pre-trial conference on a case, and then to enforce that schedule strictly. Again, the underlying aim here appears to be to reduce the likelihood of open-ended delays in the resolution of cases.

This reform, together with the existing law that gives judges discretion over how to structure their own hearings, seems consonant with another anecdotal comment that came from several of our interviews with workers' compensation lawyers: namely, that there are some broad regional differences in the nature of proceedings in Pennsylvania and that proceedings in the eastern part of the state may tend to be more aggressively adversarial and litigious than those elsewhere. According to this viewpoint, mandatory trial scheduling may have been driven primarily by pressures in the eastern part of the commonwealth. It remains to be seen what the effects of mandatory trial scheduling will ultimately be and whether those effects will be consistent across Pennsylvania.

Perhaps the best observation we can offer on these issues is that the commonwealth, having recently adopted a new reform on trial scheduling, is now in a strong position to evaluate the effects of that reform going forward, as well as the impact of the diverse serial hearing practices employed by different judges in the past. On the latter point, it is noteworthy that Pennsylvania already has survey data from each of its judges describing whether, and how, they use serial hearing procedures (Pennsylvania Department of Labor and Industry, Office of Adjudication, 2003). That kind of information could be combined with other data on dispute resolution across the commonwealth to explore performance patterns associated with serial hearings, and to investigate whether the various arguments about timeliness or cost are actually borne out in Pennsylvania. In sum, it seems likely that the issue of one-day-one-trial will continue to come up in the future: Policymakers would be well served by an analytical review of the impact of past practices and of current reforms, as a predicate to any future modifications of hearing and trial scheduling procedures in Pennsylvania.

Compromise and Release

One of the biggest statutory changes to the Pennsylvania workers' compensation system involved the incorporation of "compromise and release" agreements under Act 57. Prior to 1996, the Pennsylvania system did not have any statutory provision to support the formal, final resolution of claims through a lump-sum settlement procedure.[2] Following the reform, Pennsylvania reversed its course from foreclosing such agreements (in the putative interest of workers and the public) to becoming a state in which C&R agreements account for a very significant proportion of all benefits paid to workers on an annual basis (Torrey, 2007). According to the most recent available summary data, more than 14,000 C&R settlements were approved in Pennsylvania in the 2005/06 fiscal year, resulting in payments of more than $770 million—an amount that corresponds to approximately 29 percent of the total compensation paid in calendar year 2005 (DLI, 2007b). Notably, both the amount of money awarded through C&R on an annual basis, as well as the proportion of C&R payments in relation to total compensation paid, have continued to grow during the most recent several years for which data are available (Torrey, 2007). The adoption of the C&R procedure by Pennsylvania has also been associated with a number of systemic benefits, including accelerated resolution of cases and reduction of case backlogs, although the causal relationship between C&R and these benefits is not without ambiguity (Torrey, 2007).

---

[2]   As one commentator points out, Pennsylvania did permit *commutation* of workers' compensation claims prior to 1996, but traditional commutation required neither a final settlement agreement nor the resolution of a controversy. Instead, it involved an agreement for accelerated payment of the discounted present value of a future stream of benefits. See Torrey (2007, p. 256).

In stakeholder interviews, we heard mixed commentary on the advantages and drawbacks that have been associated with C&R. On one hand, we heard that C&R does facilitate the faster resolution of cases that should (from the perspective of both sides of the bar) be resolved quickly. We also heard that C&R complements the mediation of disputes, since C&R is the basis for a formal and final settlement of claims. On the other hand, we heard concerns that lump-sum payments may sometimes fail to cover the medical and indemnity losses that the system was intended to insure, and that some claimants may not have the sophistication or discipline to handle lump-sum payments appropriately on their own behalf. These sorts of concerns echo the traditional arguments that have been made against C&R in workers' compensation systems generally (Torrey, 2007). Other concerns about C&R expressed by a recent Pennsylvania commentator include the lack of a "bona fide dispute" requirement (i.e., that there actually be a meaningful conflict over facts or law that becomes the subject of a "compromise"); the limited standard of judicial review (which focuses only on the claimant's understanding of the C&R agreement and not on his or her best interests); and the possibility that some injured workers might settle when faced with arbitrary denials or challenges to their benefits by employers (Torrey, 2007). The same commentator described his own personal experience with C&R as a workers' compensation judge in Pennsylvania, and he indicated that the majority of claimants he encountered in reviewing C&R petitions had low incomes, were working class, and had tendered releases both for future disability payments and future medical care in connection with their C&R settlements. Perhaps troubling, he also found that only a tiny minority of claimants indicated that they were entering into C&R with the intent of using their settlements for purposes of vocational rehabilitation (i.e., ultimately to replace lost income) (Torrey, 2007). By implication, this calls into question the adequacy of those C&R settlements as direct compensation for loss of future income (or even for medical costs).

As a matter of policy, C&R has become the linchpin of Pennsylvania's efforts to promote the early resolution of workers' compensation disputes other than through litigation. And Act 147 has recently built on that same foundation, both by establishing a requirement for mandatory mediation of disputes and by creating a resolution-hearing mechanism to expedite the judicial review of C&R settlements. In light of the foregoing, two questions arise: What additional reforms, building on the C&R framework, are likely to be proposed in the future? And what effects has C&R actually had on the workers' compensation system, beyond the fact that an increasing fraction of cases in the system are now being resolved in this way? Regarding the first question, Torrey (2007) suggests that pressures for ever faster resolution of workers' compensation disputes are unlikely to abate and might well lead to proposals (for example) to delete the current statutory requirement for open hearings, as a predicate to the final confirmation of C&R settlements. Torrey argues that this kind of reform could ultimately have negative effects both for claimants and for employers and insurers, by leaving the former more vulnerable to overreaching and manipulation, and the latter more vulnerable to attempts to set aside or reopen established settlements. Implicitly, this kind of concern once again highlights the fact that speed in resolving cases is not the only criterion for success in the workers' compensation system: The performance of the system must also be judged in light of other considerations, including fundamental fairness, appropriateness of compensation, and finality of settlements.

For policymakers, C&R presents another aspect of workers' compensation policy for which additional information on system performance could be helpful in determining the appropriateness of future calls for reform. One avenue for such investigation could involve an expanded version of the more limited analysis undertaken by Torrey (2007), simply by collecting more comprehensive data on the characteristics of C&R claimants, settlements, and related proceedings throughout Pennsylvania, over a period of several years. A more ambitious analytical approach might look at the impact that C&R has had on the adequacy of settlements in actually replacing lost wages, using similar methods to those employed in previous studies of permanent partial disability in other states (Reville et al., 2005). Alternatively, policymakers might consider undertaking experimental pilot programs on a limited basis for new C&R reforms (e.g., eliminating the open hearing requirement) as a way to evaluate those sorts of reforms before enacting them into law more broadly. In any event, policymakers will likely want to fine-tune C&R proceedings over time, in order to best capture the benefits of expedited resolution of claims, while balancing that goal against continued judicial oversight and appropriate compensation. Additional data, analysis, and experimentation would likely be helpful in pursuing these ends.

Mandatory Mediation

At the same time that the Pennsylvania legislature adopted the C&R procedure in 1996, it also added a statutory provision to enable workers' compensation judges to conduct informal mediation conferences to resolve disputes. Voluntary mediation was an initial step in providing a state-supervised alternative channel for working out disputes without recourse to full litigation. In 2006, the legislature went a step further by adding a *mandatory* mediation provision to the statute. Pennsylvania law now requires that judges schedule a mediation conference early in the litigation process, barring a finding on good cause that mediation would be futile. Again, the idea here is to promote faster resolution of disputed claims and to funnel disputes toward a lower-cost resolution mechanism. The movement to strengthen mediation procedures in Pennsylvania reflected a sentiment expressed by LBFC in 2005, namely, that the commonwealth had lagged in applying alternative dispute resolution (ADR) techniques during the early 1990s, thereby contributing to higher litigation rates (LBFC, 2005). In interviews with stakeholders, we heard mixed comments about the impact of mediation. Two people noted that only a small fraction of cases had been resolved through mediation prior to 2006, that Pennsylvania judges were uneven in their aptitude at running mediations, and that it was unclear that the new mandatory provisions would change outcomes much. Another observed that mandatory mediation imposed a major cultural change on judges, with effects difficult to predict. For example, mandatory mediation could plausibly have the effect of increasing pressure on workers to compromise disputed claims, a result that might or might not be appropriate in specific instances, depending on the nature of the disputes.

It is likely premature to discuss prospects for future mediation reforms in Pennsylvania, in the absence of good information on the effects of the reforms already instituted. Recent annual reports from the Office of Adjudication make it clear that many workers' compensation judges provide mediation services, but the reports do not describe the experience across the commonwealth in terms of numbers and types of cases resolved through mediation, the nature and consistency of mediation procedures across Pennsylvania, etc. If the purpose of mediation is to resolve cases more quickly without detracting from the quality of outcomes, then policymakers should, ideally, be informed about how successful mediation has been in accomplishing that purpose. We can readily envision any number of additional reforms to mediation requirements in the future, such as modifying the legal standards for when mediation needs to take place, who can be present during the proceedings, and what the scope and powers of the mediators should be. But the logical threshold step prior to considering any of these sorts of interventions is to gather more data on current practices and outcomes, any changes that occurred in the wake of Act 147, and any systemic differences that emerge across the cases that do, and do not, settle through mediation. Without more of that kind of information, it is not at all clear what the specific aims of any future mediation reforms should actually be.

Medical Depositions Versus Reports

A narrow issue in Pennsylvania workers' compensation adjudication that has previously been subject to criticism involves reliance by the system on medical depositions, rather than on reports, in many proceedings. Both LBFC and WCRI identified the trend toward depositions in Pennsylvania as being associated with above-average medical-legal costs relative to those of other states (LBFC, 2005; Telles, Wang, and Tanabe, 2006b). Because depositions involve taking physician testimony (and, in at least some instances, permitting cross-examination), they can frequently be expensive to conduct and time-consuming to schedule. The stakeholders we interviewed on this issue expressed conflicting points of view. We heard both that the opportunity to cross-examine in medical testimony can be crucial in workers' compensation cases (and that "the right to confrontation is protected under the Pennsylvania constitution"), as well as the view that in some cases where medical issues are undisputed, reports could probably serve as a decent substitute for depositions. In this regard, it is notable that the statute currently allows for medical reports to be entered as evidence in workers' compensation cases, although in disputes involving prolonged disability, this requires consent from both parties to the litigation.[3]

In the interest of promoting medical reports as a way to reduce litigation delays, BWC formed a committee in 2002 to explore specific ways to encourage the use of reports in litigated cases. In sum, the committee (1) recommended the adoption of standardized report forms, and (2) observed some basic ambiguities regarding the constitutional status of medical reports entered as evidence (Torrey and Greenberg, 2002). Without getting deeply into technical details, these sorts of recommendations highlight the fact that the rules of evidence in workers' compensation litigation offer another potential focus for reform efforts. As it happens, the use of medical reports may be an issue for which some changes could be made without the need for modified statutory authority. On the other hand, it is also clear that the success of this type of reform would depend on convincing litigants, rather than compelling them, to depart from the standard practice of using depositions. Based on feedback from our own limited stakeholder interviews, we sense that depositions remain the preferred or default evidence mechanism for some (and perhaps most) counsel. It remains an open question whether any continuing delays and incremental costs associated with depositions would justify an effort to introduce formal legislative reforms to compel change on this issue.

Discussion and Policy Implications

Dispute resolution in the Pennsylvania workers' compensation system is a key institutional device for allowing the system to work effectively. Based on the foregoing discussion, we would like to emphasize several points. First, the dispute resolution system in itself involves a complex and highly technical set of policies and administrative mechanisms. We have focused on

---

[3]   At Sections 422(a) and (c) of the Workers' Compensation Act (Commonwealth of Pennsylvania, 1915).

a subset of major, illustrative policy issues in this chapter, based partly on input from our own stakeholder interviews and partly on the substance of legislative initiatives passed in the last decade. Certainly, other aspects of workers' compensation adjudication (such as the nature and impact of the appeals process) could also be explored as targets of reform. Nevertheless, the policy issues that we've addressed here are probably among the most important ones, as reflected both by past reforms that have modified the basic structure for resolving disputes in the commonwealth and by continuing interest among stakeholders, policymakers, and scholars in fine-tuning these aspects of the system.

Second, a consistent theme that arises in connection with dispute resolution policy in Pennsylvania involves the need for more and better data resources with which to examine the effects of different aspects of policy. Trial scheduling, C&R, and mediation are all examples of major reforms designed to improve the efficiency of resolving disputes in the workers' compensation system. But it is difficult to know what the full impact of these measures has been in the absence of detailed data on implementation, patterns of resolution in claims, and corresponding effects on timing and costs in litigation. The Office of Adjudication has already made a commendable effort to collect and publish summary data on a number of aspects of litigation in the commonwealth. More data and deeper analysis would likely be helpful to policymakers and the public in better understanding and evaluating what the impact of recent reforms has been.

Finally, we note that most of the pressure to reform dispute resolution in workers' compensation appears to derive from concerns about delays in litigation proceedings and related costs. To the extent that previously published summary data address the broad performance of the dispute resolution system, those data suggest to us that the system has been getting faster in resolving disputes over recent years and that Pennsylvania does not appear to be an outlier on measures of litigiousness and litigation costs when compared with a number of other states. Equally important, though, is the recognition that those sorts of findings on speed and cost do not represent the only important performance criteria for the system. An effective dispute resolution system needs to pursue not only efficiency but also finality, high quality outcomes, appropriate compensation, and fairness to all of the participants in the system. This is a multi-valent evaluative framework, one which is difficult to capture through currently available data. Nevertheless, policymakers will need to consider the balance among all of these dimensions in the context of any future initiatives to change the system.

CHAPTER SIX

Discussion

The primary aim of this paper has been to examine the performance of the Pennsylvania workers' compensation system across several of its major functions and to identify and explore some of the major policy issues that the system faces. This paper has also endeavored to recommend some options that the commonwealth should consider in addressing those issues in the future (see Table 6.1). Where possible, we have grounded our discussion by reviewing available evidence and published data on the recent performance of the system. Our main focus in this paper has been on several specific aspects of the system, including benefits and employer costs, safety, medical care, and dispute resolution. These are all important elements of the workers' compensation framework, but it is worth repeating that they do not exhaust the field of inquiry concerning workers' compensation policies. Most notably, we did not set out in this paper to investigate the insurance aspects of the system, even though insurance issues may present significant challenges for the future. In the course of our stakeholder interviews, for example, one person commented that the Pennsylvania workers' compensation system is confronting a broader, national problem in managing risks associated with catastrophic terrorism. Although this goes beyond the scope of our current paper to address, it is nevertheless worth acknowledging the nexus between terrorism and workers' compensation policy, because it illustrates a more general point: namely, that the workers' compensation system does not operate in a vacuum, but rather is deeply influenced by broader social trends, as well as by a number of other aspects of national and state policy.

In a related vein, we also heard several (sardonic) comments to the effect that one solution to rising medical costs in workers' compensation might be to institute a universal, single-payer health care scheme. Without commenting in detail on that specific premise, it does reflect the fact that we (and others) can readily imagine plausible, sweeping changes to the basic contours of workers' compensation in Pennsylvania. Other studies have occasionally evaluated options for major systems re-engineering, as in the context of California proposals to integrate employer-based health coverage and workers' compensation medical coverage into a unified "24-hour care" mechanism (Farley et al., 2004). Our aim in this paper has been more prosaic and focuses mainly on incremental prospects for reform, extensions of policies that have already been tried, and on ideas or concerns that were raised through our conversations with stakeholders. In general, we did not hear stakeholders express the desire for fundamental, sweeping changes in the current structure of the workers' compensation system. Instead, we heard that the system has already undergone some important changes in the last 15 years and has likely improved on some performance benchmarks. We also heard concerns about mixed effects connected with some of the enacted reforms (e.g., C&R agreements) and suggestions

Table 6.1
Summary of Policy Recommendations on Workers' Compensation

Policy Issue	Recommendation
Wage replacement	Pennsylvania policymakers should consider the adequacy of wage replacement, as well as systemic payment levels, in assessing the overall performance of the workers' compensation system.
C&R agreements	Pennsylvania should collect and aggregate more information about C&R agreements, who is entering into them, and what the major features of those agreements are. Any future proposals for additional C&R reforms, such as eliminating hearing requirements or by mandating the existence of a genuine dispute between litigating parties, should be formally evaluated on a pilot or prospective basis.
Mediation	Pennsylvania should track mediation processes and outcomes going forward, and could thereby help policymakers in reviewing any future proposals to refine or expand upon the current mediation requirements.
Injury rates	Pennsylvania should consider requesting that BLS increase its Survey of Occupational Injuries and Illnesses sample in the commonwealth, so that comparable state-level injury rates will become available.
Safety committees	Pennsylvania should seek better performance data to gauge the impact of certified safety committees on workplace injuries, as a precursor to seeking to expand the reach and influence of safety committees in the employer community.
Medical costs, quality of care, and access to care	Policymakers should continue to track measures of medical costs, and should improve the tracking of quality of care and access within the workers' compensation system, given that the pressures for medical cost containment are unlikely to diminish.
The medical fee schedule	As a precursor to any proposal to restructure the current workers' compensation medical fee schedule to harmonize it with Medicare, Pennsylvania should first undertake a detailed study of the price implications and implementation options, along the lines of a similar assessment that was performed in California in 2003.
Other reforms	With regard to other future medical policy reforms, Pennsylvania should incorporate a formal, prospective assessment of their effects on cost, quality of care, and access.

for additional, incremental policy changes and performance assessments that might be helpful in the future.

This focus on incrementalism in workers' compensation policy is consonant with the picture that emerges from aggregate performance data describing the system over recent years. Not surprisingly, total workers' compensation payments in Pennsylvania have been on the rise, but when adjusted for payroll growth, those payments were basically flat during the period between 2000 and 2004. And although average total costs on a per-claim basis rose over roughly the same period, Pennsylvania's performance on that measure nevertheless seems to compare reasonably well with that of a number of other states. Of course, cost is only one dimension of the system's performance, and data on other performance criteria, such as adequacy of indemnity benefits, are more difficult to come by. Survey findings suggest that Pennsylvania is doing reasonably well on several benchmarks concerning access to, and workers' satisfaction with, medical care. Comparative interstate data describing these sorts of outcomes, however, are very limited, as are data on safety outcomes and rates of occupational injuries. We do note that currently available data suggest that medical payments in Pennsylvania are on the rise and may be particularly important as a driver of cost growth in the future. And although limited in scope, available data also suggest that Pennsylvania may not compare strongly with other states on at least some measures of safety outcomes. Consequently, the medical and safety dimensions of workers' compensation policy may become increasingly important as targets for additional reform efforts.

One obvious question that arises, in light of this window into performance, is how emerging changes in Pennsylvania's demographic patterns and industry mix are likely to impact on the workers' compensation system. With regard to demographic patterns, recent Census bureau projections indicate that Pennsylvania's population is growing older and that the median age in the commonwealth may rise from 38 years (per data from the 2000 Census) to 42 years by 2030 (U.S. Census Bureau, 2005). Notably, previous empirical research on older workers has suggested that the likelihood of occupational injury declines with age, but that older workers may nevertheless be more likely than younger workers to suffer permanent disabilities, as well as larger wage losses, lower wage replacement rates, and more injury-related days of nonemployment (Biddle, Boden, and Reville, 2003; Burton and Spieler, 2001). These are troubling findings, given the demographic trends toward an aging workforce in Pennsylvania. Meanwhile, with regard to industry mix, projections by the Pennsylvania Center for Workforce Information and Analysis suggest that employment in non-durables manufacturing will shrink by almost 20 percent between 2004 and 2014 (Pennsylvania Center for Workforce Information and Analysis, 2007). By contrast, employment in the services and health care sectors is projected to grow significantly during the same time period. Taken together with the most recent commonwealth data showing lower rates of occupational injuries in the services sectors as compared with manufacturing (BWC Claims Management Division, 2006), the projections could imply that rates of workplace injury in Pennsylvania will decline somewhat in coming years. Whether any of these projected demographic and industry effects on workers' compensation will actually manifest, however, remains to be seen.

Perhaps the most consistent theme that emerges from the review in this paper is simply the need for broader and more robust data collection, and publication of performance results, across a number of different aspects of the Pennsylvania workers' compensation system. BWC, DLI, and the Office of Adjudication already do very significant data collection and summary analyses in connection with their annual reports and survey studies. Those efforts could be strengthened and augmented, even through some very simple steps, such as making previous years of the commonwealth's annual reports on workers' compensation available online. This notwithstanding, there remain some notable gaps in published performance data for some elements of the workers' compensation system, particularly so for data that can support comparisons between Pennsylvania and other states. Another basic step for improving the performance data and benchmarks that are currently available to policymakers would be to better leverage external data collection mechanisms (such as by expanding participation in the BLS Survey of Occupational Injuries and Illnesses). On a complementary note, the enactment of specific workers' compensation reforms (e.g., medical provider panels, C&R agreements, etc.) always invites the question whether the reforms have been successful in achieving their underlying aims. Going forward, it may make sense to institute new reforms on an experimental pilot basis, and/or to incorporate formal, prospective assessment as an essential design element in implementation. Again, this could help to provide more and better information to policymakers, both in assessing and refining the impact of new workers' compensation policies.

On a final, general note, we reiterate that the performance of the workers' compensation system, and the effectiveness of reforms thereto, cannot be evaluated solely in terms of cost. As a matter of historical motivation, it is likely accurate that concerns about cost were among the primary considerations in the legislative passage of Acts 44 and 57 during the 1990s. But at its heart, the system nevertheless continues to reflect a basic compromise between the interests of workers and employers, one designed to redress a set of injuries that would otherwise fall unfairly on workers, with invidious costs to employers and society as well. For that reason, the workers' compensation system has to be judged for what it accomplishes as well as for what it costs. Effective wage replacement, high-quality medical care, swift and impartial judicial review are all important outcomes in themselves, as well as metrics for gauging whether the money invested in workers' compensation is purchasing a product worth buying. A myopic focus on the costs of workers' compensation can lead to an odd perspective on related policies. It is, after all, fairly easy to formulate ways to cut costs—provided that we do not care about compensation, medical benefits, due process, or helping injured workers return to their jobs. By recognizing this broader spectrum of performance criteria, we reaffirm the critical importance of ongoing data collection and analysis, in order to understand how the system is really doing, while placing considerations of cost in appropriate context. We also stand in better position thereby to identify the most promising targets for reform—namely, those that align the interests of workers and employers and offer the potential to improve the system for both groups of key stakeholders.

Conclusions and Recommendations

- Currently available data suggest that benefit payments in the Pennsylvania system, adjusted for payroll growth, have been relatively flat during 2000–2004 and that Pennsylvania compares favorably with a number of other states on several measures of average costs per workers' compensation claim. Far less clear is the adequacy of wage replacement associated with Pennsylvania's indemnity benefits and how well Pennsylvania compares to other states on this criterion. *Pennsylvania policymakers should consider the adequacy of wage replacement, as well as systemic payment levels, in assessing the overall performance of the system.* Either BWC or independent researchers should be encouraged to perform analyses on the adequacy of wage replacement in the commonwealth, so that policymakers can track and understand related trends over time.

- One of the most important reforms to the Pennsylvania system over the past 15 years was the institution of compromise and release agreements, which allow claimants and insurers to negotiate final, lump-sum settlements in discharge of workers' compensation liability. Nearly a third of the total benefits paid by the system in 2005 were disbursed through C&R agreements. Here again, though, the impact of C&R settlements on adequacy of wage-replacement benefits, long-term vocational outcomes, and medical care for injured workers is not well understood. *Ideally, the commonwealth should collect and aggregate more information about C&R agreements, who is entering into them, and what the major features of those agreements are.* Future studies of wage-replacement adequacy in Pennsylvania should also look specifically at the impact of C&R, as compared with the traditional payment of claims. *Finally, any future proposals for additional C&R reforms, such as eliminating hearing requirements or mandating the existence of a genuine dispute between litigating parties, should be formally evaluated on a pilot or prospective basis.*

- New requirements for dispute mediation, instituted in 2006, are among the most recent reforms to the Pennsylvania system. Under the revised law, all workers' compensation claims that enter litigation must be mediated, except where a judge makes a finding on good cause that mediation would be futile. Given the newness of the requirements for mediation, however, there is currently no information on the effects of the mandate, on the nature and volume of cases resolved in the commonwealth through mediation, or on whether mediation produces materially different outcomes than adjudication across otherwise similar cases. *Pennsylvania stands in good position to track these kinds of measures going forward, and could thereby help policymakers in reviewing any future proposals to refine or expand on the current mediation requirements.*

- Rates of workplace injuries in Pennsylvania fell substantially between 1996 and 2005, according to aggregated workers' compensation data published by the commonwealth. Interstate comparisons of occupational injury rates are hampered, however, by differences in underlying definitions and methods for compiling data across the states. Notably, the Bureau of Labor Statistics (BLS) fields an annual Survey of Occupational Injuries and Illnesses, which estimates industry-specific injury rates both nationally and for 42 states, not including Pennsylvania. *The commonwealth should consider requesting that BLS increase its survey sample in Pennsylvania, so that comparable state-level injury rates will become available.*

- One of Pennsylvania's major initiatives to promote workplace safety involves encouraging employers to adopt certified safety committees, by providing a 5-percent discount on workers' compensation insurance premiums for participating employers. Uptake of certified safety committees within the employer community has been modest, however, and the limited safety performance data on the committees that are currently available through PCRB are only suggestive, but not conclusive, that the state certification program has had a beneficial effect. *Pennsylvania should seek better performance data to gauge the impact of certified safety committees on workplace injuries, as a precursor to any effort to expand the reach and influence of safety committees in the employer community.* More broadly, the commonwealth should consider new ways to make the financial benefits to employers of improved safety performance more transparent and more salient, throughout the employer community.

- Medical payments represent the part of aggregate workers' compensation payments that are growing most rapidly in Pennsylvania (and across the nation). And although Pennsylvania, when compared with a number of other states, has lower average medical costs on a per-claim basis, general trends toward growth in medical costs remain a subject of concern. Meanwhile, only limited performance data are currently being collected by the commonwealth describing access and quality of care within the Pennsylvania system, and interstate comparisons and benchmarking on those sorts of parameters are very limited. *Policymakers should continue to track measures of medical cost, and should improve the tracking of quality of care and access within the workers' compensation system, given that the pressures for medical cost containment are unlikely to diminish.*

- One aspect of the workers' compensation medical framework that has occasionally been criticized is the medical fee schedule, which in turn is based on the Medicare schedule from the early 1990s. Medicare fees have since been revised in ways not reflected by the Pennsylvania fee schedule, thereby giving rise to concerns about administrative burdens, as well as the potential for perverse incentives to providers that might undercut the aim of containing costs. We note that any proposed reform to the Pennsylvania fee schedule, particularly if intended to emulate current fee rates under Medicare, would likely involve highly technical details in the transition, as well as significant groups of winners and losers within the provider community. *As a precursor to any such proposal, we recommend that the commonwealth undertake a detailed study of the price implications of, and implementation options for, revising the medical fee schedule, along the lines of a similar assessment that was performed in California in 2003 (Wynn, 2003).*

- Pennsylvania has implemented several other important policies for containing workers' compensation medical costs since 1993, including provider panel requirements and utilization review oversight. Both of these mechanisms could be refined or expanded on in the future, and as of fall 2007, the commonwealth was reviewing a set of proposed regulations to update and clarify the current framework for utilization review. *We suggest that any future reforms to these policies incorporate a formal, prospective assessment of their ultimate effect on costs, as well as on health care quality and access.* This kind of performance information could help policymakers in evaluating the successfulness of the policies, as well as in refining them going forward.

Bibliography

Actuarial and Technical Solutions, Inc., "Workers Compensation State Rankings: Manufacturing and Industry Costs and Statutory Benefit Provisions, 2006 Edition," Ronkonkoma, N.Y.: Actuarial and Technical Solutions, Inc., 2006.

Belton, Sharon E., Richard. A. Victor, and Te-Chun Liu, *Comparing Outcomes for Injured Workers in Nine Large States*, Cambridge, Mass.: Workers Compensation Research Institute, 2007.

Biddle, Jeff, Leslie I. Boden, and Robert T. Reville, "Older Workers Face More Serious Consequences from Workplace Injuries," *Health and Income Security for an Aging Workforce*, Vol. 5, 2003.

Blum, Florence, and John F. Burton, Jr., "Workers' Compensation Benefits: Frequencies and Amounts in 2002," *Workers' Compensation Policy Review*, Vol. 6, No. 5, September–October, 2006, pp. 3–27.

Bureau of Economic Analysis, "Regional Economic Information System," 2007. As of February 7, 2008:
http://www.bea.gov/regional/docs/reis2005dvd.cfm

Bureau of Labor Statistics, "Workplace Injuries and Illnesses in 2001," 2002.

———, "Census of Fatal Occupational Injuries (CFOI)—Current and Revised Data," Web page, February 5, 2008. As of February 7, 2008:
http://www.bls.gov/iif/oshcfoi1.htm

———, "Local Area Unemployment Statistics," Web page, undated. As of January 25, 2008:
http://www.bls.gov/lau/

Burton, John F., and Emily A. Spieler, "Workers' Compensation and Older Workers," in Peter B. Budetti, Richard V. Burkhauser, Janice M. Gregory, and Allan H. Hunt, eds., *Ensuring Health and Income Security for an Aging Workforce* (proceedings of the National Academy of Social Insurance, Washington, D.C., January 26–27, 2000), Kalamazoo, Mich.: W. E. Upjohn Institute, 2001.

BWC Claims Management Division—*see* Pennsylvania Bureau of Workers' Compensation, Claims Management Division.

Cocchiarella, Gunnar, and B.J. Anderson, ed., *Guides to the Evaluation of Permanent Impairment*, Chicago, Ill: American Medical Association, 2001.

Commonwealth of Pennsylvania, Workers' Compensation Act, P.L. 736, No. 338, June 2, 1915.

———, Act 44, P.L. 190, No. 44, July 2, 1993.

———, Act 57 of 1996, P.L. 530, No. 57, June 24, 1996.

———, "Proposed Rulemaking on Medical Cost Containment," *Pennsylvania Bulletin*, Vol. 36, No. 23, Notice 2139, June 10, 2006a. As of January 25, 2008:
http://www.pabulletin.com/secure/data/vol36/36-23/1056.html

———, Act 147, P.L. 1362, No. 147, November 9, 2006b.

———, Pennsylvania Code, Title 34, Section 129.1005, Committee Responsibilities, 2007a.

———, Pennsylvania Statutes, Title 77, Section 511, Schedule of Compensation for Total Disability, 2007b.

———, Pennsylvania Statutes, Title 77, Section 1038.1, Accident and Illness Prevention Services, 2007c.

—————, Pennsylvania Statutes, Title 77, Section 1038.2, Certification of Safety Committee, 2007d.

Connolly, Ceci, "Insurer Agrees to Pay Doctors $198 Million; Deal Hailed as Victory over Managed Care," *Washington Post*, July 12, 2005, p. A02.

DeBernardo, Heidi J., "Pennsylvania Workers' Compensation Law: An Examination of Key Changes Made to Supersedeas Proceedings by Act 57 of 1996," *Duquesne University Law Review*, Vol. 35, No. 3, spring 1997, pp. 881–895.

DLI—*see* Pennsylvania Department of Labor and Industry.

Donabedian, Avedis, *Explorations in Quality Assessment and Monitoring, Vol. 1: The Definition of Quality and Approaches to Its Assessment*, Ann Arbor, Mich.: Health Administration Press, 1980.

—————, *Explorations in Quality Assessment and Monitoring, Vol. 2: The Criteria and Standards of Quality*, Ann Arbor, Mich.: Health Administration Press, 1982.

Eccleston, Stacey M., Dongchun Wang, and Xiaoping Zhao, *The Anatomy of Workers' Compensation Medical Costs and Utilization: Technical Appendix, 5th Edition*, Cambridge, Mass.: Workers Compensation Research Institute, 2005a.

—————, *The Anatomy of Workers' Compensation Medical Costs and Utilization in Pennsylvania, 5th Edition*, Cambridge, Mass.: Workers Compensation Research Institute, 2005b.

Eccleston, Stacey M., and Xiaoping Zhao, *Benchmarking the 2004 Pennsylvania Workers' Compensation Medical Fee Schedule*, Cambridge, Mass.: Workers' Compensation Research Institute, 2004.

Farley, Donna O., Michael D. Greenberg, Christopher Nelson, and Seth A. Seabury, *Assessment of 24-Hour Care Options for California*, Santa Monica, Calif.: RAND Corporation, MG-240-ICJ, 2004. As of January 22, 2008:
http://www.rand.org/pubs/monographs/MG280/

Gray, Wayne B., and Carol Adaire Jones, "Are OSHA Health Inspections Effective? A Longitudinal Study in the Manufacturing Sector," *Review of Economics and Statistics*, Vol. 73, No. 3, 1991, pp. 504–508.

Gray, Wayne B., and John M. Mendeloff, "The Declining Effects of OSHA Inspections on Manufacturing Injuries: 1979 to 1998," Cambridge, Mass.: National Bureau of Economic Research, Working Paper 9119, 2002.

Greenberg, Andrew E., "Workers' Compensation Reform: Legislative Update," presented at the Pennsylvania Self-Insurers' Association Fall Workshop, Reading, Pa., October 7, 2005. As of February 7, 2008:
http://www.chartwelllaw.com/publish/A1010.pdf

Hunt, H. Allan, "Benefit Adequacy in State Workers' Compensation Programs," *Social Security Bulletin*, Vol. 65, No. 4, 2003/2004, pp. 24–30.

Illinois Workers' Compensation Commission, *FY 2005 Annual Report*, Chicago, Ill., 2006.

Indiana University of Pennsylvania, "Pennsylvania SHA Consultation Program," Web page, undated. As of January 24, 2008:
http://www.hhs.iup.edu/sa/OSHA/index.htm

Latzko, David A., "Industry Mix, Wages, and the Divergence of County Income in Pennsylvania," *Review of Urban and Regional Development Studies*, Vol. 13, No. 2, July 2001, pp. 110–122.

LBFC—*see* Pennsylvania General Assembly Legislative Budget and Finance Committee.

McGlynn, Elizabeth A., Steven M. Asch, John Adams, Joan Keesey, Jennifer Hicks, Alison DeCristofaro, and Eve A. Kerr, "The Quality of Health Care Delivered to Adults in the United States," *New England Journal of Medicine*, Vol. 348, No. 26, June 26, 2003, pp. 2,635–2,645.

Mendeloff, J. M. and Wayne B. Gray, "Inside the Black Box: How Do OSHA Inspections Lead to Reductions in Workplace Injuries?" *Law & Policy*, Vol. 27, No. 2, 2005, pp. 219–237.

Miller, N. W., "Workers' Compensation Laws Undergo Significant Change," *Pennsylvania Medicine*, Vol. 97, No. 2, 1994, pp. 52–53.

New York State Workers' Compensation Board, *Annual Report of the New York State Workers' Compensation Board*, Albany, N.Y., 2005.

Nuckols, Teryl, "The Value of High Quality Medical Care in Workers' Compensation," *IAIABC Journal*, Vol. 44, No. 1, spring 2007, pp. 15–35.

Oregon Department of Consumer and Business Services, "Oregon Workers' Compensation Premium Rate Ranking, Calendar Year 2004," Salem, Ore., 2005.

———, "Biennial Report on the Oregon Workers' Compensation System," Salem, Ore., 2006.

Pennsylvania Bureau of Workers Compensation, Claims Management Division, "Pennsylvania Work Injuries and Illnesses: 2003," Harrisburg, Pa., 2004.

———, "Pennsylvania Work Injuries and Illnesses: 2004," Harrisburg, Pa, 2005.

———, "Pennsylvania Work Injuries and Illnesses: 2005," Harrisburg, Pa., 2006.

Pennsylvania Center for Workforce Information and Analysis, "Industry & Employment Projections," Web page, 2007. As of February 7, 2008:
http://www.paworkstats.state.pa.us/analyzer/

Pennsylvania Compensation Rating Bureau, "Analysis of Experience Under the Pennsylvania Certified Safety Committee Program," Philadelphia, Pa., 2006.

———, "Proposal C-352 Loss Cost Filing, Exhibit 8," Philadelphia, Pa., 2007.

Pennsylvania Department of Labor and Industry, *2002 Workers' Compensation Medical Access Study: Executive Overview*, Harrisburg, Pa., 2003.

———, *2003 Workers' Compensation Medical Access Study: Executive Overview*, Harrisburg, Pa., 2004.

———, *2004 Workers' Compensation Medical Access Study: Executive Overview*, Harrisburg, Pa.: Pennsylvania Department of Labor and Industry, 2005.

———, *2005 Workers' Compensation Medical Access Study: Executive Overview*, Harrisburg, Pa.: Pennsylvania Department of Labor and Industry, 2006a.

———, *Pennsylvania Workers' Compensation and Workplace Safety: Annual Report Fiscal Year 2004/05*, Harrisburg, Pa., 2006b.

———, "Health and Safety Division Introduces HandS System," Web page, 2007a. As of January 24, 2008:
http://www.dli.state.pa.us/landi/cwp/view.asp?a=138&q=231472

———, *Pennsylvania Workers' Compensation and Workplace Safety: Annual Report Fiscal Year 2005/06*, Harrisburg, Pa., 2007b.

———, "Return-to-Work: A Model for Pennsylvania Business and Industry," Web page, 2007c. As of January 24, 2008:
http://www.dli.state.pa.us/landi/cwp/view.asp?a=312&q=212054

———, "WorkSAFE PA Initiative," Web Page, 2007d. As of January 24, 2008:
http://www.dli.state.pa.us/landi/cwp/view.asp?a=144&q=208344

Pennsylvania Department of Labor and Industry, Office of Adjudication, "Office of Adjudication Judgebook: Practice and Procedure Before Workers' Compensation Judges," Web page, 2003. As of January 22, 2008:
http://www.dli.state.pa.us/landi/cwp/view.asp?a=138&q=196465

Pennsylvania General Assembly, House Resolution No. 660, 2004.

Pennsylvania General Assembly Legislative Budget and Finance Committee, "Pennsylvania Workers' Compensation System Compared to Nearby States," Harrisburg, Pa., 2005.

Public Law 91-596, Occupational Health and Safety Act of 1970, December 29, 1970.

Reinke, Derek, and Mike Manley, "2006 Oregon Worker's Compensation Premium Rate Ranking Summary," Salem, Ore.: Oregon Department of Consumer and Business Services, 2006.

Reno, Virginia P., and Ishita Sengupta, *Pennsylvania Workers' Compensation Benefits and Coverage, 2004*, Workers' Compensation Brief No. 8, Washington, D.C.: National Academy of Social Insurance, 2006. As of January 23, 2008:
http://www.nasi.org/usr_doc/NASI_Workers_Comp_2004.pdf

Reville, Robert T., Leslie I. Boden, Jeff E. Biddle, and Christopher Mardesich, *An Evaluation of New Mexico Workers' Compensation Permanent Partial Disability and Return to Work*, Santa Monica, Calif.: RAND Corporation, MR-1414-ICJ, 2001. As of January 22, 2008:
http://www.rand.org/pubs/monograph_reports/MR1414/

Reville, Robert T., Seth A. Seabury, Frank W. Neuhauser, John F. Burton, Jr., and Michael D. Greenberg, *An Evaluation of California's Permanent Disability Rating System*, Santa Monica, Calif.: RAND Corporation, MG-258-ICJ, 2005. As of January 22, 2008:
http://www.rand.org/pubs/monographs/MG258/

Rosenman, Kenneth D., Alice Kalush, Mary Jo Reilly, Joseph C. Gardiner, Mathew Reeves, and Zhewui Luo, "How Much Work-Related Injury and Illness Is Missed by the Current National Surveillance System?" *Journal of Occupational and Environmental Medicine*, Vol. 48, No. 4, April 2006, pp. 357–365.

Sengupta, Ishita, Virginia P. Reno, and John F. Burton, Jr., *Workers' Compensation: Benefits, Coverage, and Costs, 2004*, Washington, D.C.: National Academy of Social Insurance, 2006. As of January 23, 2008:
http://www.nasi.org/usr_doc/NASI_Workers_Comp_2004.pdf

———, *Workers' Compensation: Benefits, Coverage, and Costs, 2005*, Washington, D.C.: National Academy of Social Insurance, 2007. As of January 23, 2008:
http://www.nasi.org/usr_doc/NASI_Workers_Comp_2005_Full_Report.pdf

Stark, Karl, "Judge's Ruling Resumes Pay Plan: The Settlement Between the Philadelphia Orthopedic Society and Blue Cross Is to Bring $40 Million-Plus to Doctors," *Philadelphia Inquirer*, April 26, 2004, p. F01.

Telles, Carol A., Dongchun Wang, and Ramona P. Tanabe, "A Comparison of System Features: 13 States," Cambridge, Mass.: Workers Compensation Research Institute, 2006a.

———, *CompScope Benchmarks, 6th Edition: The DataBook*, Cambridge, Mass.: Workers Compensation Research Institute, 2006b.

———, *CompScope Benchmarks, 6th Edition: Technical Appendix*, Cambridge, Mass.: Workers Compensation Research Institute, 2006c.

———, *CompScope Benchmarks for Pennsylvania, 6th Edition*, Cambridge, Mass.: Workers' Compensation Research Institute, 2006d.

Torrey, David B., "Compromise Settlements Under State Workers' Compensation Acts: Law, Policy, Practice, and Ten Years of the Pennsylvania Experience," *Widener Law Journal*, Vol. 16, No. 2, 2007, pp. 199–469.

Torrey, David B., and Andrew E. Greenberg, *Workers' Compensation: Law and Practice*. St. Paul, Minn.: Thomson West, 2002.

U.S. Census Bureau, Population Division, "Interim State Population Projections," Washington, D.C., 2005.

Victor, Richard A., *Evidence of Effectiveness of Policy Levers to Contain Medical Costs in Workers' Compensation*, Cambridge, Mass.: Workers Compensation Research Institute, 2003.

Victor, Richard. A., Peter S. Barth, and Te-Chun Liu, *Outcomes for Injured Workers in California, Massachusetts, Pennsylvania, and Texas*, Cambridge, Mass.: Workers Compensation Research Institute, 2003.

Weil, David, "If OSHA Is So Bad, Why Is Compliance So Good?" *RAND Journal of Economics*, Vol. 27, No. 3, autumn 1996, pp. 618–640.

Wynn, Barbara O, *Adopting Medicare Fee Schedules: Considerations for the California Workers' Compensation Program*, Santa Monica, Calif.: RAND Corporation, MR-1776-ICJ, 2004. As of January 22, 2008:
http://www.rand.org/pubs/monograph_reports/MR1776/